BASIC NOTES IN PSYCHIATRY

Revised Edition

Previous books by the same author

Levi, M.I. (1987) *MCQs for the MRCPsych Part I* (Lancaster: MTP Press)

Levi, M.I. (1988) *MCQs for the MRCPsych Part II* (Lancaster: Kluwer Academic Publishers)

Levi, M.I. (1988) *SAQs for the MRCPsych Part II* (Lancaster: Kluwer Academic Publishers)

Levi, M.I. (1992) *PMPs for the MRCPsych Part II* (Lancaster: Kluwer Academic Publishers)

BASIC NOTES IN PSYCHIATRY

Revised Edition

Dr Michael I Levi
MB, BS, MRCPsych

with a Foreword by
Dr A Margo, FRCPsych
Consultant Psychiatrist, Goodmayes Hospital, Ilford, Essex, UK

KLUWER ACADEMIC PUBLISHERS
DORDRECHT / BOSTON / LONDON

Distributors

for the United States and Canada: Kluwer Academic Publishers, PO Box 358, Accord Station, Hingham, MA 02018-0358, USA
for all other countries: Kluwer Academic Publishers Group, Distribution Center, PO Box 322, 3300 AH Dordrecht, The Netherlands

British Library Cataloguing in Publication Data is available.

ISBN 0-7923-8990-5

Copyright

First edition 1989
Revised edition 1992

Published in the United Kingdom by Kluwer Academic Publishers, PO Box 55, Lancaster, UK.

Kluwer Academic Publishers BV incorporates the publishing programmes of D. Reidel, Martinus Nijhoff, Dr W. Junk and MTP Press.

Printed in Great Britain by Hartnolls Limited, Bodmin, Cornwall.

Contents

Foreword

The novice in psychiatry requires a skeletal framework which he can clothe progressively with more detail and sophisticated understanding. Without structure the naive in the subject must fail to orientate through to a clearer conceptualization of key and relevant issues in psychiatry today. To allow for the acquisition of basic concepts, review and revision, any provisional framework should of necessity be concise and unpretentious. In this book Dr. Michael Levi has succeeded in creating a good starting point for the retention of new knowledge, which can then be built on through diverse reading and clinical experience.

A. Margo, FRCPsych
Consultant Psychiatrist

Introduction

The purpose of writing this book is to provide a concise summary of general adult psychiatry in the form of notes. I have based these notes on what is generally regarded to be the most easily readable and evenly written textbook[1] for the MRCPsych examination.

The book is intended to have wide readership – particularly among junior hospital psychiatrists, general practitioners and medical students. In addition, the book will also be useful to psychiatric nurses, psychiatric social workers and clinical psychologists.

Reference

1. Gelder, M., Gath, D. and Mayou, R. (1989). *Oxford Textbook of Psychiatry – Second Edition* (Oxford: Oxford Medical Publications)

Preface to the Revised Edition

Following the popularity of my first edition, I was encouraged to write this edition for junior hospital psychiatrists, general practitioners and medical students.

I have taken note of the various comments of users of the first edition. The section on formulation in the first chapter has been considerably revised and several additions have been made to the management sections of chapters four, six and seven, to keep up with the pace of modern treatment methods in psychiatry.

Acknowledgements

I wish to thank Dr A. Margo for writing the Foreword to this book. Thanks once again to Dr J.M. Brewis of Kluwer Academic Publishers for giving me the opportunity of publishing my fourth book. A special thank you must yet again go to Mr S. Ogrodzinski of Duphar Laboratories Limited who helped me to secure the publication of my material. Many thanks to Dr H.N. Ball for his advice on the first chapter regarding formulation. Finally, thank you again to my parents for their support.

CHAPTER 1

The History, Mental State Examination and Formulation

As in any branch of medicine, psychiatry begins with taking a good history and examining the patient. The history is very similar in format to that taken in general medicine, while the mental state examination is something very particular to psychiatry. Having done both of these, it is then necessary to provide a formulation – i.e. a summary of the case presented in an integrated or synthesized fashion. This chapter deals with, in turn, the history, the mental state examination and the formulation.

THE HISTORY

Age/Marital Status/Occupation

Source of referral

1. **PC/HPC** (Presenting complaint/history of the presenting complaint)
   Principal symptoms or complaints and their duration; associated disturbance in appetite, weight, sleep and sexual drive; effects on patient's ability to cope socially or with work.

2. **PPH** (Past psychiatric history)
   Previous hospital admissions with psychiatric illness. Treatment given. How well did patient remain in between admissions?

3. **PMH/PSH** (Past medical history/past surgical history)
   Previous hospital admissions with physical illness or for operations.

4. **FH** (Family history)
   a. **Mother and father** – current age, or if dead, age at death and cause of death; occupations.
   b. **Sisters and brothers** – names, ages, marital status, occupation.
   c. **FPH** (Family psychiatric history) – history of any psychiatric illness in the family.

   d. **FMH** (Family medical history) – history of any physical illness in the family.
   e. **Current relationships** – with parents, siblings and other relatives.

5. **PH** (Personal history) **Born and bred**
   a. **Birth** – any prematurity or low birth weight; any difficulties during delivery.
   b. **Preschool development** – any delay in achieving milestones; any separation from parents; relationships with parents, siblings, other children and adults at this age.
   c. **School** – age of starting and finishing school; type of school attended; academic qualifications; relationships with pupils and teachers.
   d. **Occupations** – chronological list of jobs; if multiple changes, enquire about the reasons; relationships with workmates and superiors.
   e. **Psychosexual history** – age of onset of puberty; first steady relationship; first sexual intercourse; if married, age at marriage and age of spouse at marriage; any psychiatric or physical illness in spouse; relationship with spouse; if children, give chronological list of their names, age and sex; any psychiatric or physical illness in children; relationship with children.

6. **Smoke** – current and past smoking habits.

7. **Drink** – current and past drinking habits.

8. **Drugs** – drugs, medicines or tablets patient is currently taking; any abuse of illicit drugs (e.g. cannabis, amphetamines, opiates).

9. **Allergies** – any known allergies.

10. **Social circumstances** – current type of residence (e.g. flat, house); composition of household.

11. **Forensic history** – any trouble with the law or police; any convictions.

12. **PMP** (Premorbid personality) – the patient's personality before first admission to hospital with psychiatric illness.
   a. **Relationships** – few friends or many.
   b. **Character** – outgoing or reserved.

c. **Mood** – cheerful or gloomy; steady or changeable.
d. **Leisure activities** – preference for company or solitude.

THE MENTAL STATE EXAMINATION

1. **Appearance and behaviour** –
   a. **Dress and self-care** – tidy or dishevelled, well-groomed or unkempt; describe actual clothes.
   b. **Manner** – hostile or helpful, aggressive or amiable.
   c. **Posture and movement** – tense or relaxed, overactive or slowed-up.
   d. **Appropriateness** – in touch with surroundings or listening to hallucinatory voices.

2. **Speech** – pressure or poverty of speech; spontaneous or hesitant; coherent or incoherent; neologisms.

3. **Mood** –
   a. Subjective report.
   b. Depression or elation.
   c. Anxiety, irritability, fear or hostility.
   d. Incongruity or blunting of affect.
   e. Suicidal ideation.

4. **Thought** –
   a. **Content** – worries or preoccupations; obsessions or delusions; passivity phenomena; persecutory ideation.
   b. **Form** – pressure or poverty of thought; thought blocking; loosening of associations or flight of ideas or perseveration; interpretation of proverbs.

5. **Perception** – hallucinations; illusions; depersonalization or derealization.

6. **Cognition** –
   a. **Orientation** – in time, place, person and age.
   b. **Attention and concentration** – subjective report, days of week backwards (DOWB) or months of year backwards (MOYB); serial sevens test or serial threes test; digit span forwards and backwards (5 to 7 numbers).

c. **Memory** – subjective report and:
   i. **Immediate memory** – name and address, immediate recall; Babcock sentence; digit span (as above).
   ii. **Recent memory** – name and address, 5 minute recall; menu of most recent meal.
   iii. **Remote memory** – personal events recalled from several years ago; assessed in the history.

d. **Grasp** – Prime Minister of UK; President of USA; reigning monarch of UK; any item of current affairs.

7. **Insight** –
   a. Does the patient consider himself ill in psychological terms?
   b. Does the patient feel in need of treatment?

THE FORMULATION

1. **Introduction** – salient features of history (positives and negatives).

2. **Current mental state examination** –
   Label psychopathological features.

3. **Diagnosis** –
   Support with reasons from mental state examination and history.

4. **Differential diagnosis** –
   a. The diagnostic hierarchy is useful in deciding this –
      1. Personality disorders.
      2. Neuroses.
      3. Paranoid states.
      4. Affective disorders.
      5. Schizophrenia.
      6. Organic disorders.

      A high-priority condition (e.g. organic disorders) can be accompanied by the symptoms of a low-priority condition (e.g. neuroses), but only the high-priority condition need be diagnosed.
   b. There should be a maximum of two conditions to be considered in the differential diagnosis – to indicate you have synthesized the case.
   c. Each condition should be supported with reasons from the mental state examination and history.

5. **Aetiology** –
Predisposing, precipitating and maintaining factors

6. **Investigations** –
   a. More information: Speak to informants (e.g. spouse, relatives, friends); speak to general practitioner; obtain reports from other agencies (e.g. school, employers); old case notes.
   b. Further assessments:
      1. **Physical** – full physical examination, blood tests, urine tests, X-rays, EEG, ECG.
      2. **Social** – social worker's report; family interview.
      3. **Psychological** – psychometry (i.e. assessment of general intelligence, personality and neuropsychological status by a clinical psychologist).
      4. **Others** – observations by nursing staff; occupational therapy assessments (e.g. assessment of daily living).

7. **Management** –
   a. Short-term: Inpatient versus outpatient; ? compulsory order; immediate physical treatment; contributions by nursing staff, social worker and occupational therapist.
   b. Long-term:
      1. **Physical** – subsequent physical treatment with drugs and ECT (electroconvulsive therapy).
      2. **Social** – part played by other members of the multidisciplinary team (e.g. social worker, community psychiatric nurse); social provisions or supports; family involvement; rehabilitation.
      3. **Psychological** – supportive psychotherapy versus formal psychotherapy versus brief interviews to assess progress; behaviour therapy (including cognitive behaviour therapy, relaxation training and anxiety management training).

8. **Prognosis** –
   a. State whether poor or good with reasons, e.g. good prognosis because of acute onset and presence of a precipitating factor.
   b. Consider the prognosis both for this episode and in the long term.

CHAPTER 2

The Symptoms and Signs of Mental Illness

As in any branch of medicine, making a diagnosis in psychiatry is based on:

I. **Eliciting the symptoms** – by asking the patient about the presenting complaint and the history of the presenting complaint.

II. **Eliciting the signs** – by examining the mental state of the patient for psychopathological features.

The framework for eliciting the symptoms and signs is the history and mental state examination, as detailed in the first chapter. The purpose of this chapter is to describe the various psychopathological features which may be seen in the mental state examination. The diagnostic significance of each feature will be pointed out in the various chapters to follow on general adult psychiatry.

I. **Appearance and behaviour** –
   1. **Appearance** – mood may be expressed in the form of:
      a. **Appearance** – facial expression, posture.
      b. **Manner** – response to others.
      c. **Motility** – degree and form of movements.

   2. **Behaviour** – there are several motor disorders of general behaviour –
      a. **Echolalia** – repetition by the patient of the interviewer's words or phrases.
      b. **Echopraxia** – imitation by the patient of the interviewer's movements.
      c. **Stereotypy** – regular, repetitive non goal-directed movement (i.e. purposeless).
      d. **Mannerism** – abnormal, repetitive goal-directed movement (i.e. of some functional significance).

e. **Chorea** – random, jerky movements, resembling fragments of goal-directed behaviour (i.e. semi-purposeful).
f. **Athetosis** – slow, writhing, semi-rotatory movements.
g. **Waxy flexibility** – the patient's limb can be placed in an awkward posture and remain fixed in position over a long period, despite asking the patient to relax (also called catalepsy).
h. **Mitmachen** – the patient's body can be placed in any posture, despite asking the patient to resist all movements. When released, the patient returns to the resting position (cf. waxy flexibility).
i. **Mitgehen** – an extreme form of mitmachen in which the patient will move in any direction with very slight pressure.
j. **Gegenhalten (opposition)** – the patient will oppose attempts at passive movement with a force equal to that being applied (cf. mitmachen).
k. **Negativism** – an extreme form of gegenhalten, in which there is an apparently motiveless resistance to suggestion or attempts at movement.
l. **Automatic obedience** – the patient does whatever the interviewer asks of him irrespective of the consequences.
m. **Ambitendence** – the patient begins to make a movement but, before completing it, starts the opposite movement.
n. **Stupor** – a state of more or less complete loss of activity with no reaction to external stimuli, although the patient is conscious.
o. **Perseveration** – the senseless repetition of a previously requested movement, i.e. the repetition of a motor response after the stimulus is withdrawn.

II. **Speech** –

1. **Pressure of speech** – rapid and copious speech, as thoughts crowd into the patient's mind in quick succession.
2. **Poverty of speech** – slow and sparse speech, as thoughts enter the patient's mind only occasionally.
3. **Neologisms** – the patient uses words or phrases invented by himself.
4. **Mutism** – the total loss of speech.

III. **Mood** –

1. **Incongruity of affect (inappropriate affect)** – the mood is not in keeping with the mood that would ordinarily be expected, e.g. the patient may laugh when told about a bereavement.
2. **Blunting of affect (flattening of affect)** – sustained emotional indifference or diminution of emotional response.

    N.B. Mood and affect are often used interchangeably to mean the same thing. Technically, however, there is a difference between them –

    Affect – a short-lived disorder of emotion.

    Mood – a sustained disorder of emotion.

IV. **Thought** –

1. **Content** –
    a. **Obsessions** – recurrent, persistent thoughts, impulses, or images that the patient regards as absurd and alien (ego-alien), while recognizing them as the product of his own mind (ego-syntonic). Attempts are made (at least early on) to resist or ignore them. Frequently the obsessions are of an aggressive or sexual nature.

    b. **Delusion** – a false belief with the following characteristics: firmly held despite evidence to the contrary; out of keeping with the person's educational and cultural background; content often bizarre; often infused with a sense of great personal meaning.

    c. **Passivity phenomena** – the individual experiences interference with, or outside control of, his thinking, feeling, perception or behaviour. This is due to the apparent disintegration of boundaries between the self and the surrounding world. There are several types:

    i. **Thought insertion** – the experience of thoughts being put into the mind by some external force.

    ii. **Thought withdrawal** – the experience of thoughts being taken out of the mind by some external force.

    iii. **Thought broadcasting** – the experience that others can 'read' the individual's thoughts as they are 'broadcast' from his mind.

    iv. **'Made' volition** – the experience that free will is removed and behaviour is controlled by some external force.

    N.B. Technically passivity phenomena are disorders of the possession of thought. However, by convention they are included under disorders of the content of thought.

2. **Form** –
   a. **Pressure of thought** – ideas arise in unusual variety and abundance, and pass through the mind rapidly.
   b. **Poverty of thought** – the patient has only a few ideas, which lack variety and abundance, and pass through the mind slowly.
   c. **Thought blocking** – the experience of the patient's mind going entirely blank in the middle of a train of thought.
   d. **Loosening of associations** – loss of the normal structure of thinking. Muddled and illogical conversation that cannot be clarified by further enquiry. It can take several forms –
      i. **Knight's move (derailment)** – a transition from one topic to another with no logical relationship between the two topics and no evidence of links between these topics as seen in flight of ideas (see below).
      ii. **Word salad (verbigeration)** – disruption of both the connection between topics and the finer grammatical structure of speech.
      iii. **Talking past the point (vorbeireden)** – the patient seems always about to get near to the matter in hand, but never quite reaches it.
   e. **Flight of ideas** – the patient's thoughts and conversation move quickly from one topic to another, so that one train of thought is not completed before another appears. The links between these rapidly changing topics are understandable, because they occur in normal thinking, i.e. rhyming, punning, clang associations and responding to distracting cues in the immediate surroundings.
   f. **Perseveration** – the persistent and inappropriate repetition of the same thoughts. In response to a series of different questions the patient gives the correct answer to the first, but continues to answer subsequent questions with the answer to the first question.

   N.B. Technically pressure of thought, poverty of thought and thought blocking are disorders of the stream of thought. However, by convention they are included under disorders of the form of thought.

V. **Perception** –

1. **Hallucinations** – perceptions which arise in the absence of any external stimulus.
2. **Illusions** – distortions of perceptions of real objects.
3. **Depersonalization** – a change in self-awareness such that the person feels unreal.
4. **Derealization** – a change in self-awareness such that the environment feels unreal.

VI. **Cognition** –

1. **Age disorientation** – the patient can correctly give his date of birth and the current date, but gives a gross underestimate of his current age.
2. **Serial sevens test** – subtraction of serial sevens from 100.
3. **Serial threes test** – subtraction of serial threes from 40.
4. **Digit span** – a series of digits repeated forwards and backwards. Begin with 5 numbers and build up to 7.
5. **Babcock sentence** – 'one thing a nation must have to become rich and great is a large secure supply of wood'.

CHAPTER 3

Personality Disorders

DEFINITION

Deeply ingrained, maladaptive patterns of behaviour; recognizable in adolescence or earlier; continuing throughout most of adult life; either the patient or others have to suffer; there is an adverse effect on the individual or society.

EPIDEMIOLOGY

More commonly diagnosed in:

1. Age group 18–35.
2. Male sex.
3. Lower social class.

CLINICAL FEATURES

I. **Affective personality disorder** – 3 groups –
   1. **Depressive personality disorder** – always low in spirits; persistently gloomy view of life; brood about misfortunes; worry unduly; strong sense of duty; little capacity for enjoyment.
   2. **Hyperthymic personality disorder** – habitually cheerful and optimistic; striking zest for living; poor judgement; periods of irritability when aims frustrated.
   3. **Cyclothymic personality disorder** – alternate between being low in spirits and being cheerful and optimistic; gloomy defeatist approach to life as mood changes from hyperthymic to depressive; reduced energy.

II. **Anankastic personality disorder** (obsessional personality disorder) – lack of adaptability to new situations; high moral standards; humourless approach to life; miserly; sensitivity to criticism; indecision; emotionally constricted.

III. **Antisocial personality disorder** (sociopathic or asocial personality disorder) – impulsive actions; lack of guilt; failure to make loving relationships; failure to learn from adverse experiences.

IV. **Asthenic personality disorder** (passive or dependent personality disorder) – weak-willed; unduly compliant; lack vigour; lack self-reliance; avoid responsibility; little capacity for enjoyment.

V. **Avoidant personality disorder** – hypersensitive to rejection; low self-esteem; unwillingness to enter into relationships; desire for acceptance.

VI. **Borderline personality disorder** – unstable relationships; undue anger; variable moods; chronic boredom; doubts about personal identity; intolerance of being left alone; self-injury; impulsive behaviour that is damaging to the person.

VII. **Explosive personality disorder** – instability of mood with outbursts of anger and violence; no other difficulties in relationships (cf. antisocial personality disorder).

VIII. **Histrionic personality disorder** – self-dramatization; a self-centred approach to personal relationships; a craving for excitement and novelty.

IX. **Narcissistic personality disorder** – grandiose sense of self-importance; preoccupation with fantasies of unlimited success, power and intellectual brilliance; attention demanding but show little warm feeling in return; exploitative but do not give favours in return.

X. **Paranoid personality disorder** – strong sense of self-importance; suspicious; hypersensitive; cold affect; argumentative and stubborn.

XI. **Passive–aggressive personality disorder** – passive resistance to demands for adequate performance; stubborn; intentionally inefficient.

XII. **Schizoid personality disorder** – introspective; prone to engage in an inner world of fantasy rather than take action; lack of emotional warmth and rapport; self-sufficient and detached; aloof and humourless; incapable of expressing tenderness or affection; shy; often eccentric; insensitive; ill-at-ease in company.

XIII. **Schizotypal personality disorder** – superstitious ideas; an interest in telepathy and clairvoyance; unrealistic (magical) thinking; odd forms of speech.

AETIOLOGY

I. **Genetic** – no satisfactory evidence about the genetic contribution to personality disorders.

II. **Body build (Kretschmer)** –
   1. Pyknic (stocky and rounded) build – related to cyclothymic personality disorder.
   2. Asthenic (lean and narrow) build – related to schizoid personality disorder.

III. **Psychoanalytic theory** – serious difficulty in passing through the anal stage of development will result in anankastic personality disorder.

IV. **Childhood influences on personality development** – maternal separation has been proposed as a cause of antisocial personality disorder.

DIFFERENTIAL DIAGNOSIS

I. **Exclude any organic disorders** – e.g. focal or diffuse organic brain disease, epilepsy, alcohol or drug abuse.

II. **Exclude any functional psychiatric illness** – e.g. schizophrenia, affective disorders, neuroses.

MANAGEMENT

I. **Physical** –
   1. **Short-term** – anxiolytic drugs or neuroleptics may be given for short periods at times of unusual stress.
   2. **Long-term** – neuroleptics may be helpful in paranoid and schizotypal personality disorders.

II. **Social** – supervision and support are often beneficial. This can be given by a doctor, social worker or psychiatric nurse.

III. **Psychological** – for the majority, psychotherapy is not indicated. Group psychotherapy is more helpful than individual psychotherapy. Confrontative psychotherapy is more helpful than interpretative psychotherapy. Psychotherapy is least likely to help people with antisocial personality disorders, although some are helped by large group psychotherapy in the form of a therapeutic community – in such a unit, the patients meet several times a day for group discussions, in which each person's behaviour and feelings are examined by the other group members.

IV. **General measures** –
1. The treatment plan aims to bring about limited changes in the patient's circumstances, so that he has less contact with situations that provoke his difficulties, and more opportunity to develop the assets in his personality.
2. Admission to hospital should be avoided whenever possible, but may be necessary for short periods of crisis.

PROGNOSIS

I. Personality disorders tend to become rather less disordered as the patient grows older.

II. Patients with antisocial personality disorders over the age of 45 present fewer problems of aggressive behaviour than patients under the age of 45. However, their problems of personal relationships tend to persist.

CHAPTER 4

Neuroses

ANXIETY NEUROSES

Definition

Various combinations of psychological and physical manifestations of anxiety, not attributable to real danger and occurring either in attacks (panic disorder) or as a persisting state (generalized anxiety disorder). Other neurotic features may be present (obsessional or hysterical symptoms) but do not dominate the clinical picture.

Epidemiology

I. Often begins in early adult life – but may occur for the first time in middle age.

II. More common among women.

III. The most common neurotic disorder with a prevalence rate of 3% – if minor depressive disorders are excluded from the neuroses.

Clinical features

I. **Psychological symptoms and signs** – fearful anticipation; irritability; a feeling of restlessness; sensitivity to noise; repetitive worrying thoughts; difficulty in concentration; subjective report of poor memory.

II. **Physical symptoms** –
   1. **Respiratory symptoms** – difficulty in inhaling (cf. difficulty in expiration in asthma); feeling of constriction in the chest; overbreathing and its consequences – feeling of weakness; feeling of breathlessness; faintness; numbness; tinnitus; tingling in hands, feet and face; dizziness; headache; carpopedal spasms; precordial discomfort.
   2. **Cardiovascular symptoms** – feeling of discomfort or pain over the heart; palpitations; throbbing in the neck; awareness of missed beats.

3. **Gastrointestinal symptoms** – excessive wind caused by aerophagy; borborygmi; difficulty in swallowing; dry mouth; epigastric discomfort; frequent or loose motions.
4. **Genito-urinary symptoms** – increased frequency and urgency of micturition; increased menstrual discomfort and amenorrhoea (in women); failure of erection; lack of libido.
5. **Neurological symptoms (related to CNS)** – tinnitus; dizziness; prickling sensations; blurring of vision.
6. **Musculo-skeletal symptoms** – aching and stiffness – especially in back and shoulders; trembling hands – impairs delicate movements; headache.
7. **Sleep disturbance** – difficulty getting off to sleep; after eventually falling asleep, patient wakes intermittently; often unpleasant dreams experienced; occasionally 'night terrors' experienced – in which patient wakes suddenly feeling intensely fearful.

Aetiology

I. **Genetic** – evidence for a genetic aetiology provided by:
   1. **Family studies** – prevalence rate of the disorder in relatives of patients with anxiety neuroses is 15% (cf. prevalence rate of disorder in general population of 3%).
   2. **Twin studies** (Slater and Shields) – 50% of monozygotic (MZ) twins concordant for anxiety neuroses, cf. only 2.5% concordance in dizygotic (DZ) twins.

II. **Biochemical and endocrine investigations** –
   1. Increased secretions of adrenaline and noradrenaline in anxious patients.
   2. Higher lactate levels after exercise in patients with anxiety neuroses, cf. normal subjects.

III. **Psychoanalytic theory** – anxiety is experienced for the first time during the process of birth (primary anxiety). The child is overwhelmed by stimulation at the very moment of separation from its mother. This may explain why maternal separation can cause anxiety neuroses.

IV. **Learning theory** – explains the tendency to develop excessive anxiety in terms of an inherited predisposition that is:
   1. Reflected in undue lability of the autonomic nervous system.
   2. Detected by measures of neuroticism.

Differential diagnosis

I. Exclude organic disorders in which anxiety symptoms occur – presenile and senile dementia; alcohol and drug abuse; thyrotoxicosis; phaeochromocytoma; hypoglycaemia.

II. Exclude functional psychiatric illnesses in which anxiety symptoms occur – depressive illness; schizophrenia.

Management

I. **Physical** –
   1. **Benzodiazepines** – provide symptomatic relief of anxiety in the short term (should not be prescribed for more than a few weeks), e.g. diazepam; dose range 5 mg b.d. to 10 mg t.d.s.
   2. **Tricyclic antidepressants** – appropriate when medication has to be prolonged beyond the few weeks for which benzodiazepines are prescribed. Non-addictive, cf. benzodiazepines; effective due to their anxiolytic properties; may have more specific effects on autonomic reactivity in panic disorder e.g. imipramine.
   3. **5-HT reuptake inhibitors** – e.g. fluvoxamine. Some evidence for usefulness in panic disorders.
   4. **β-Blockers** – limited use in treating anxiety neuroses in which palpitations are the most troublesome symptom.
   5. **Monoamine oxidase inhibitors (MAOIs)** – some evidence for usefulness in panic disorders due to anxiolytic properties.
   6. **Psychosurgery** – reserved for cases of chronic, intractable, incapacitating anxiety, unresponsive to other measures.

II. **Social** – social intervention aimed at current situational stresses.

III. **Psychological** –
   1. **Psychotherapy** – for most brief anxiety neuroses, reassurance and counselling with the doctor are usually sufficient, i.e. anxiolytic drugs need not be prescribed.
   2. **Behaviour therapy** –
      a. **Relaxation training** – this procedure uses a simple system of exercises intended to bring about relaxation of individual groups of skeletal muscles and to regulate breathing. Such simple relaxation is effective in reducing mild to moderate anxiety but not severe anxiety.
      b. **Anxiety management training (AMT)** – may be more effective than simple relaxation; 2 stages –

i. Verbal cues and mental imagery are used to arouse anxiety.
ii. The patient is trained to reduce this anxiety by relaxation, distraction and reassuring self-statements.

Prognosis –

I. Anxiety neuroses of recent onset – most recover quickly.
II. Anxiety neuroses lasting more than six months – 80% are present three years later despite efforts at treatment.
III. Poor prognosis is associated with – agitation; derealization; syncopal episodes; suicidal ideas; hysterical features.
IV. Patients who complain of physical symptoms are less easy to treat than those who recognize the emotional basis for their disorder.

PHOBIC ANXIETY NEUROSES

Definition –

Neurotic states with an abnormally intense dread of certain objects or specific situations which would not normally have that effect. The dread is accompanied by a strong wish to avoid the feared objects or situations.

Epidemiology –

I. **Simple phobic neuroses** (include animal phobias) –
   1. Onset in childhood for animal phobias; onset in early adult life for other specific phobias.
   2. More common among women.

II. **Agoraphobia** –
   1. Onset usually between ages 15–35.
   2. More common among women.

III. **Social phobic neuroses** –
   1. Onset usually between ages 17–30.
   2. Equally common in men and women.

Clinical features –

I. **Simple phobic neuroses** –
   1. Some specific object or situation causes the person unreasonable anxiety, e.g. spiders, dogs, heights, thunderstorms, darkness.

2. There are three components –
    a. Anxiety symptoms identical to those of any other anxiety state.
    b. Anxious thoughts usually in anticipation of situations the person may have to encounter.
    c. The habit of avoiding situations that provoke anxiety.

II. **Agoraphobia** –
1. Strictly a fear of open spaces – but often used for a fear of:
    a. Shops and supermarkets.
    b. Buses and trains.
    c. Crowds.
    d. Any place that cannot be left suddenly without attracting attention, e.g. a seat in the middle of a row in the theatre.
2. The anxiety symptoms are identical to those of any other anxiety state. However, the associated anxious thoughts are characteristically centred on ideas of fainting or losing control.
3. As the condition progresses, the patient increasingly avoids the places or situations that provoke anxiety, so that only a few local shops can be reached.
4. In the most severe cases, the patient cannot leave the house at all – this condition is known as the housebound housewife syndrome.
5. Certain other non-phobic symptoms are common among agoraphobic patients – depersonalization, depression, obsessions.

III. **Social phobic neuroses** –
1. A fear of, and habit of avoiding, situations in which the individual may be observed by other people (e.g. restaurants, dinner parties, public transport). Also a fear that the individual may behave in a manner that will be humiliating or embarrassing (e.g. blushing, shaking).
2. The anxiety symptoms are identical to those of any other anxiety state.
3. The anxious thoughts are usually in anticipation of situations the person may have to encounter.
4. Certain other non-phobic symptoms occur among patients with social phobic neuroses – depersonalization, depression, obsessions (less frequent than in agoraphobic patients).

Aetiology

I. **Simple phobic neuroses** –
Psychoanalytic theory – the manifest fear is the symbolic representation of an unconscious conflict, i.e. the simple phobic neuroses represent some other source of anxiety that has been excluded from consciousness by repression and displacement.

II. **Agoraphobia** –
1. **Psychoanalytic theory** – when unconscious conflicts are not allowed direct expression because of repression, this may be transformed by displacement into phobias.
2. **Learning theory** – agoraphobia develops as a series of conditioned fear responses with learned avoidance.

III. **Social phobic neuroses** – The main reason why a patient should develop a social phobia rather than some other kind could be:
1. The circumstances in which the first episode of acute anxiety was experienced.
2. General lack of self-confidence in social encounters.

Differential diagnosis –

I. **Simple phobic neuroses** – seldom present difficulties of differential diagnosis.

II. **Agoraphobia** – exclude: anxiety neuroses; social phobic neuroses; depressive disorders; paranoid states.

III. **Social phobic neuroses** – exclude: social inadequacy; personality disorders; anxiety neuroses; depressive disorders; schizophrenia.

Management

I. **Physical** –
1. **Anxiolytic drugs** – provide some immediate relief of phobic symptoms in the short term.
2. **Antidepressant drugs** –
   a. Effective because of anxiolytic properties.
   b. MAOIs – reduce agoraphobic symptoms, but there is a high relapse rate when drugs are stopped.
   c. Imipramine – some clinicians consider this tricyclic antidepressant to be the treatment of choice for agoraphobia.

II. **Social** – lasting improvement requires attention to the accompanying avoidance behaviour. In cases of recent onset – the patient should be encouraged to make determined efforts to go out more.

III. **Psychological** – behaviour therapy is usually necessary once avoidance behaviour has become established –

1. Simple phobic neuroses of an object or situation encountered readily – treatment by exposure is used, i.e. the patient is exposed to the object or situation being avoided.
2. Simple phobic neuroses of an object or situation not encountered readily (e.g. thunderstorms) – systematic desensitization in imagination is used –
   a. Patients are required to imagine the anxiety-provoking situations vividly, starting with those that evoke little fear and progressing through carefully planned stages (a 'hierarchy') until the patient habituates and the avoidance response is extinguished.
   b. At each state anxiety is neutralized by relaxation training.
3. Agoraphobia – the treatment of choice is programmed practice
   a. This combines exposure to actual (cf. imagined) anxiety-provoking situations with measures to control any anxiety felt in these situations (relaxation training and AMT).
   b. The patients are trained to overcome avoidance behaviour in a planned way, and practice is carried out for at least an hour every day.
4. Social phobic neuroses – cognitive behaviour therapy is used in which exposure to feared situations is combined with anxiety management training.

Prognosis

I. **Simple phobic neuroses** – among adults, severe cases have usually persisted since childhood and continued for many years.

II. **Agoraphobia** – cases that have lasted for one year usually change little over the next five years.

III. **Social phobic neuroses** – cases that have lasted for one year usually change little over the next five years; but many improve gradually over a longer period.

OBSESSIVE COMPULSIVE NEUROSES

Definition

I. **Obsessions** – see Chapter 2.

II. **Compulsions** – the motor component of an obsessional thought.

Epidemiology

I. Onset is most commonly in early adult life.

II. Equally common among men and women.

III. Prevalence rate of 0.05%.

Clinical features

I. **Obsessions** – can occur in several forms:
   1. **Obsessional thoughts** – repeated and intrusive words or phrases, which are usually upsetting to the patient, e.g. violent, sexual and blasphemous themes.
   2. **Obsessional ruminations** – repeated worrying themes of a more complex kind, e.g. about the world ending.
   3. **Obsessional doubts** – repeated themes expressing uncertainty about previous actions, e.g. whether or not the person turned off a gas tap that might cause a fire.
   4. **Obsessional impulses** – repeated urges to carry out actions that are usually dangerous, aggressive or socially embarrassing, e.g. to shout obscenities in church.
   5. **Obsessional phobias** – obsessional thoughts with a fearful content, e.g. 'I must have AIDS'; or obsessional impulses that lead to anxiety and avoidance, e.g. the impulse to stab someone with a knife and the consequent avoidance of knives.

II. **Compulsions** –
   1. Also known as compulsive rituals.
   2. A compulsion is usually associated with an obsession as if it has the function of reducing the distress caused by the obsession, e.g. obsessional thoughts that the hands are contaminated with faecal matter are often followed by a handwashing compulsion.

III. **Obsessional slowness** – usually the result of obsessional doubts or compulsive rituals.

Aetiology

I. **Genetic** – some evidence for a genetic aetiology is provided by:
   1. **Family studies** – disorder occurs in 5–7% of the parents of patients with obsessive compulsive neuroses, cf. a prevalence rate of 0.05% in the general population.
   2. **Twin studies** – concordance of the disorder in MZ twins is 50–80%; cf. concordance in DZ twins of 25%.

II. **Organic factors** – some evidence for organic brain disease is provided by the frequency of obsessional symptoms in patients after the epidemic of encephalitis lethargica.

III. **Premorbid personality** – 70% of patients with obsessive compulsive neuroses have premorbid anankastic personality traits – cleanliness, orderliness, rigid, checking.

IV. **Psychoanalytic theory (Freud)** –
   1. Obsessional symptoms result from repressed impulses of an aggressive or sexual nature.
   2. Obsessional symptoms occur as a result of regression to the anal stage of psychosexual development.

V. **Learning theory** – suggests that obsessional thoughts occurring with rituals are the equivalent of avoidance responses.

Differential diagnosis

Exclude other disorders in which obsessional symptoms occur: anxiety neuroses; phobic anxiety neuroses; depressive disorders; schizophrenia; organic disorders.

Management

I. **Physical**
   1. **Anxiolytic drugs** – provide some short-term symptomatic relief. Should not be prescribed for more than a few weeks duration.
   2. **Small doses of a neuroleptic or tricyclic antidepressant** – of value when anxiolytic treatment is needed for more than the few weeks that anxiolytic drugs are prescribed.
   3. **Clomipramine** – it has been reported that this tricyclic antidepressant has a specific action against obsessional symptoms.
   4. **5-HT reuptake inhibitors** – e.g. fluvoxamine. This has also been used to treat patients with obsessive compulsive neuroses.

5. **Psychosurgery** – leucotomy is indicated in severe cases of chronic, incapacitating illness when all other methods have failed.

II. **Social** – obsessional patients often involve other family members in their rituals. In planning treatment it is essential to interview relatives and encourage them to adopt a firm but sympathetic attitude to the patient.

III. **Psychological** –
1. **Psychotherapy** – supportive psychotherapy can benefit patients by providing continuing hope.
2. **Behaviour therapy** –
   a. Obsessional thoughts occurring with rituals – exposure and response prevention i.e. by exposing the patient to those situations previously evoking checking behaviour and persuading the patient to refrain from carrying out the rituals. With persistence, the rituals and the distress subsequently diminish. The accompanying obsessional thoughts usually improve as well.
   b. Obsessional thoughts occurring without rituals – thought stopping. Patient arrests the obsessional thoughts by arranging a sudden intrusion, e.g. snapping an elastic band on the wrist.

Prognosis

I. Two-thirds of cases improve by the end of one year.

II. Cases lasting more than one year usually run a fluctuating course, with periods of partial or complete remission lasting a few months to several years.

III. Poor prognosis is associated with:
1. Anankastic personality traits.
2. Continuing stressful events in patient's life.
3. Severe symptoms.

HYSTERIA

Definition

I. Hysterical dissociation – an apparent dissociation between different mental activities.

II. Hysterical conversion – the term stems from Freud's theory that mental energy can be converted into certain physical symptoms.

Epidemiology

I. Onset usually before the age of 35.

II. Probably more common among women.

III. More common in lower social classes.

Clinical features

I. **Hysterical dissociation** – the major dissociative reactions are:
   1. Psychogenic amnesia.
   2. Psychogenic fugue (wandering).
   3. Somnambulism (sleepwalking).
   4. Multiple personality – sudden alternations between two patterns of behaviour, each of which is forgotten by the patient when the other is present.

II. **Hysterical conversion**: 'classic' conversion symptoms are:

1. Paralysis.	5. Aphonia.
2. Fits.	6. Anaesthesia.
3. Blindness.	7. Abdominal pain.
4. Deafness.	8. Disorders of gait.

III. **Primary gain** – anxiety arising from a psychological conflict is excluded from the patient's conscious mind.

IV. **Secondary gain** – the symptoms of hysteria usually confer some advantage on the patient, e.g. the attention of others.

V. **'Belle indifference'** – less than the expected amount of distress often shown by patients with hysterical symptoms.

VI. **There are no demonstrable organic findings.**

Aetiology

I. **Genetic** genetic aetiology unlikely since:
   1. **Family studies** – incidence among first-degree relatives of about 5% is higher than in the general population. However, this level most likely reflects family learning.

2. **Twin studies** (Slater) – in a sample of 12 MZ twins and 12 DZ twins, none were concordant for hysteria.

II. **Premorbid personality** – 12–21% of patients with hysteria have premorbid histrionic personality traits (see Chapter 3).

III. **Psychoanalytic theory (Freud)** –
1. Hysterics suffer from the effects of emotionally charged ideas lodged in the unconscious at some time in the past.
2. Symptoms are explained as the combined effects of repression and the 'conversion' of psychic energy into physical channels.

Differential diagnosis

I. **Exclude organic brain disease** – for example:
1. Dementia.
2. Cerebral tumour.
3. General paralysis of the insane (GPI).
4. Multiple sclerosis.
5. Complex, partial seizures (temporal lobe epilepsy).

II. **Exclude histrionic personality disorder.**

III. **Exclude malingering** – particularly among prisoners and military servicemen.

Management

I. **Physical** – abreaction:
1. Brought about by an intravenous injection of small amounts of sodium amytal.
2. In the resulting state, the patient is encouraged to relive the stressful events that provoked the hysteria, and to express the accompanying emotions.

II. **Social** –
1. **For acute cases lasting up to a few weeks** – treatment by reassurance and suggestion is usually appropriate, together with immediate efforts to resolve any stressful circumstances that provoked the reaction.
2. **General approach** – to focus on the elimination of factors that are reinforcing the symptoms, and on the encouragement of normal behaviour.

III. **Psychological** – psychotherapy
   1. Patients with hysteria usually respond well to exploratory psychotherapy concerned with their past life.
   2. They often produce striking memories of childhood sexual behaviour and other problems apparently relevant to dynamic psychotherapy.
   3. However, such ideas should not be explored at length since this may lead to over-dependence.

Prognosis

I. Cases of hysteria of recent onset – recover quickly.

II. Cases of hysteria that last longer than one year are likely to persist for many years more.

HYPOCHONDRIASIS

Definition

A neurotic disorder in which the conspicuous features are the patient's excessive concern with his health in general, in the integrity and functioning of some part of his body or, less frequently, his mind.

Epidemiology – more common among:

I. Elderly.
II. Men.
III. Lower social classes.
IV. Those closely associated with disease.

Clinical features –

I. **Pain** – common sites are:
   1. Right iliac fossa.
   2. Lower lumbar region.
   3. Head.

II. **Worries about bladder function.**

III. **Complaints about appearance** – especially the shape of the breasts, nose or ears.

IV. **Complaints about sweating or body odour.**

V. **Cardiovascular symptoms** –
   1. Dyspnoea.
   2. Left-sided chest pain.
   3. Palpitations.
   4. Worries about blood pressure.

VI. **Gastrointestinal symptoms** –
   1. Acid regurgitation.
   2. Biliousness.
   3. Nausea.
   4. Bad taste in mouth.
   5. Abdominal pain.
   6. Flatulence.
   7. Dysphagia.

Aetiology

Psychoanalytic theory –

I. Hypochondriasis is an expression of anal eroticism.

II. Hypochondriasis is a defence against psychosis.

Differential diagnosis

Exclude: personality disorders; anxiety neuroses; depressive disorders; schizophrenia; organic disorders – dementia.

Management

I. **Physical** – some advocate a trial of tricyclic antidepressants in all patients.

II. **Social** – search for meaning of symptoms in social/family setting, where appropriate. Exercise caution where symptoms serve powerful defensive purposes.

III. **Psychological** – supportive measures are the mainstay of treatment. Patients should be educated over the role of psychological factors in the symptoms.

Prognosis

I. More chronic and established cases – poor prognosis.

II. Cases associated with anxiety neuroses or depressive disorders – better prognosis.

CHAPTER 5

Paranoid States

CLASSIFICATION

I. **Simple paranoid state** – A paranoid condition that is not associated with a primary organic, schizophrenic or affective disorder, in which delusions, especially of being influenced, persecuted or treated in some special way, are the main symptoms. The delusions are of a fairly fixed, elaborate and systematized kind.

II. **Paranoia** – A permanent and unshakeable delusional system, developing insidiously in a person in middle or late life. The delusional system is encapsulated, hallucinations are absent and personality is intact. The patient can often go on working, and his social life may sometimes be maintained fairly well.

III. **Paraphrenia** – The late onset of systematized delusion, with prominent hallucinations, and preservation of personality and intellect.

IV. **Induced psychosis (Folie à deux)** – A paranoid delusional system which appears to have developed in a person as a result of a close relationship with another person who already has an established and similar delusional system. The delusions are nearly always persecutory.

V. **Special paranoid conditions** –
   1. **Othello syndrome** –
      a. **Essential feature** – a delusional belief that the marital partner is being unfaithful.
      b. **This may be accompanied by other delusions** – that the spouse is trying to poison the patient, plotting against him, infecting him with venereal disease, or taking away his sexual capacities.
      c. **Behaviour** – intensive seeking for evidence of partner's infidelity, e.g. by examining sexual organs, underwear or bed-linen for signs of sexual secretions. The patient has the desire to extract a confession from the spouse. This may

lead to severe aggression and murder.

d. **Mood** – mixture of anger, apprehension, irritability and misery.

e. **Epidemiology** – more common among men.

f. **Prognosis** – often poor.

2. **De Clerambault's syndrome** –

   a. Essential feature – a delusional belief that another person (the object), often of unattainably higher social status, loves the patient (the subject) intensely.

   b. The subject is usually a single woman.

   c. The subject believes she has been specially chosen by the object, and that it was not she who made the initial advances.

   d The subject is convinced that the object cannot be happy or a complete person without her.

   e. The subject believes that the object is unable to reveal his love to her.

   f. The subject may be importunate and disrupt the object's life.

   g. After rejection by the object, the subject's feelings may turn to hatred.

3. **Capgras' syndrome** –

   Essential feature – illusion de Sosies: a delusion in which a patient sees a familiar person and believes him to have been replaced by an imposter, who is an exact double of the original person.

4. **Fregoli's syndrome** –

   Essential feature – Fregoli's illusion: a delusion in which a patient recognizes a number of people as having different appearances, but believes that they are all a single persecutor in disguise.

AETIOLOGY

I. **Paranoia** –

   1. Cases are never, or extremely rarely, encountered.
   2. Psychoanalytic theory – associated with the ego-defence mechanisms projection and splitting.

II. **Paraphrenia** – condition best regarded as paranoid schizophrenia of late onset and good prognosis.

II. **Induced psychosis** – psychoanalytic theory – over-identification with psychotic person in a submissive over-dependent personality.

III. **Othello syndrome** –
  1. Usually associated with personality disorders or neuroses. Also associated with: depressive disorders; schizophrenia; organic disorders – e.g. alcoholism, drug abuse.
  2. Psychoanalytic theory –
    a. Projection of own desires for infidelity.
    b. Projection of repressed homosexuality.
    c. The result of other feelings of inadequacy.

V. **De Clerambault's syndrome** –
  1. Usually associated with paranoid schizophrenia. Also associated with: affective disorders; organic disorders.
  2. Psychoanalytic theory – If 'pure' form (i.e. not associated with any other disorder): projection of denied, narcissistic self-love.

VI. **Capgras' syndrome** –
  1. Usually associated with affective disorders or schizophrenia. Rarely associated with organic disorders.
  2. Psychoanalytic theory – ambivalent attitude to the person implicated.

VII. **Fregoli's syndrome** – Usually associated with schizophrenia.

MANAGEMENT

I. **Simple paranoid state** –
  1. **Physical** –
    a. Symptoms are sometimes relieved by antipsychotic medication, e.g. chlorpromazine, haloperidol, trifluoperazine, thioridazine.
    b. Choice of drug and dosage depend on:
      i. Age of patient.
      ii. Physical condition of patient.
      iii. Degree of agitation.
      iv. Response to previous medication.
    c. Commonest cause of relapse – non-compliance with medication because patients suspect medication will harm them. It may then be necessary to prescribe a long-acting

(depot) preparation, e.g. fluphenazine decanoate (Modecate).

2. **Social** – The psychiatrist should strive to maintain a good relationship with the patient. He or she should show compassionate interest in the patient's beliefs, but without condemning them or colluding in them.
3. **Psychological** – Psychological support, encouragement and assurance.

II. **Induced psychosis** –

1. **Physical** – Treat the psychotic member, if identifiable.
2. **Social** – It is usually necessary to advise separation of the affected people. This sometimes leads to the disappearance of the delusional state, improvement being more likely in the recipient than the inducer.
3. **Psychological** – Supportive psychotherapy and family therapy are often indicated.

III. **Othello syndrome** –

1. **Physical** –
   a. Treatment of any underlying disorder.
   b. In cases where underlying diagnosis is uncertain – phenothiazines, (e.g. chlorpromazine) may be beneficial.
2. **Social** – Geographical separation from partner often advisable.
3. **Psychological** –
   a. **Psychotherapy** –
      i. Given to patients with personality disorders or neuroses.
      ii. Aims to reduce tensions by allowing the patient and spouse to ventilate feelings.
   b. **Behaviour therapy** – encouraging the partner to produce behaviour that reduces jealousy, e.g. refusal to argue or counter-aggression.

IV. **De Clerambault's syndrome** –

1. Treatment of any underlying disorder.
2. If 'pure' form – very resistant to physical treatment and psychotherapy.

V. **Capgras' syndrome** – Treatment of any underlying disorder.

VI. **Fregoli's syndrome** – Treatment of any underlying disorder.

CHAPTER 6

Affective Disorders

DEFINITION

Disorders characterized by mood disturbance (inappropriate depression or elation). Usually accompanied by abnormalities in thinking and perception arising out of the mood disturbance.

CLASSIFICATION

I. **Bipolar affective disorders** – Recurring attacks of both mania and depression.

II. **Unipolar affective disorders** – Recurring attacks of depression only.

III. **Mixed affective states** – Cases where manic and depressive symptoms occur simultaneously.

EPIDEMIOLOGY

I. **Age** – depressive disorders:
   1. Women – highest prevalence rate between 35 and 45 years.
   2. Men – prevalence rate increases with age.

II. **Sex** –
   1. Bipolar affective disorders – equally common among men and women.
   2. All depressive disorders – twice as common in women.

III. **Social class** – More common in social classes I, II and V.

IV. **Marital status** – More common among the divorced or separated.

V. **Prevalence rate** – 3–4% of the general population.

CLINICAL FEATURES

A. Depressive disorders –

I. **Biological features of depression –**

1. **Sleep disturbance –**
   a. Characteristically early morning wakening (middle insomnia) – occurs 2–3 hours before the patient's usual time. He does not fall asleep again, but lies awake feeling unrefreshed with depressive thinking.
   b. Also onset insomnia (initial insomnia) – delay in falling asleep.
   c. Some depressed patients sleep excessively (cf. waking early) – but still feel unrefreshed on waking.
2. **Change in appetite –**
   a. Characteristically loss of appetite.
   b. Less commonly increased appetite.
3. **Change in weight –**
   a. Characteristically loss of weight.
   b. Less commonly increased weight.
4. **Change in psychomotor activity –**
   a. Characteristically psychomotor retardation (slowed up).
   b. Sometimes agitation.
5. **Diurnal variation in mood –**
   a. Characteristically worse in the morning.
   b. Sometimes worse in the evening.
6. **Loss of interest in work and pleasure activities.**
7. **Loss of energy and fatigue.**
8. **Loss of libido.**
9. **Change in bowel habit** – constipation.
10. **Change in menstrual cycle** – amenorrhoea.

II. **Appearance –**

1. Neglected dress and grooming.
2. Facial features –
   a. Turning downwards of corners of mouth.
   b. Vertical furrowing of centre of brow.
3. Reduced rate of blinking.
4. Reduced gestural movements.
5. Shoulders bent, head inclined forwards, direction of gaze downwards. **N.B.** Some patients maintain a smiling exterior while depressed.

III. **Speech** –
1. Poverty of speech.
2. Hesitancy – long delay before questions are answered.

IV. **Mood** –
1. One of misery.
2. Qualitatively different from normal unhappiness.
3. 'Autonomous' – i.e. loss of reactivity to circumstances.
4. Anxiety and irritability also occur.

V. **Thought** –
1. **Morbid thoughts** –
   a. **Concerned with the past** – often take form of unreasonable guilt and self-blame about minor matters, e.g. feeling guilty about past trivial acts of dishonesty.
   b. **Concerned with the present** –
      i. The patient sees the unhappy side of every event.
      ii. He thinks he is failing in everything he does and that other people see him as a failure.
      iii. He no longer feels confident, and discounts any success as a chance happening for which he can take no credit.
   c. **Concerned with the future** –
      i. Ideas of hopelessness – the patient expects the worst.
      ii. Often accompanied by the thought that life is no longer worth living for and that death would come as a welcome release.
      iii. May progress to thoughts of, and plans for, suicide.
2. **Poverty of thought.**

VI. **Psychotic features of depression** –
1. **Delusions** –
   a. Delusions concerned with themes of worthlessness, guilt, ill-health, poverty, e.g. a patient with hypochondriacal delusions (i.e. delusions of ill-health) may be convinced that he has cancer.
   b. Persecutory delusions, e.g. the patient may believe that other people are about to take revenge on him. Typically the patient accepts the supposed persecution as something he has brought upon himself.
2. **Hallucinations** –
   a. Usually second person auditory hallucinations – voices

addressing repetitive words and phrases to the patient. The voices confirm the patient's ideas of worthlessness, e.g. 'you are an evil man; you should die', or make derisive comments, or urge the patient to take his own life.

b. A few patients experience visual hallucinations, sometimes in the form of scenes of death and destruction.

VII. **Cognition** –

1. Impaired attention and concentration.
2. Poor memory.

VIII. **Physical symptoms** –

1. Aching discomfort anywhere in the body.
2. Increased complaints about any pre-existing physical disorder.

IX. **Other psychiatric symptoms** –

1. Phobic symptoms.
2. Obsessional symptoms.
3. Hysterical symptoms.
4. Hypochondriacal preoccupations.
5. Depersonalization.

B. Mania (hypomania) –

I. **Biological features of mania** –

1. **Sleep disturbance** – often reduced, but no fatigue. Patient wakes early feeling lively and energetic. Often, he gets up and busies himself noisily to the surprise of other people.
2. **Change in appetite** – increased appetite. Food may be eaten greedily with little attention to conventional manners.
3. **Change in weight** – weight loss due to overactivity.
4. **Change in psychomotor activity** – psychomotor acceleration (speeded up).
5. **Diurnal variation in mood** – though not with the regular rhythm characteristic of depressive disorders.
6. **Increased drive in work and pleasure activities.**
7. **Increased energy without fatigue.**
8. **Increased libido** – behaviour may be uninhibited. Women sometimes neglect precautions against pregnancy.

II. **Appearance and behaviour** –

1. Clothing – bright colours and ill-assorted choice of garments.
2. Untidy and dishevelled appearance.

3. Overactivity – if persistent may lead to physical exhaustion.
4. Excessive activity in risk-taking pursuits; indiscretion socially.

III. **Speech** – pressure of speech.

IV. **Mood** –
1. One of euphoria with infectious gaiety.
2. May be interrupted by brief episodes of depression.
3. Anger and irritability also occur.

V. **Thought** –
1. Expansive ideas – patient believes that his ideas are original, his opinions important, and his work of outstanding quality.
2. Pressure of thought.
3. Flight of ideas.

VI. **Psychotic features of mania** –
1. **Delusions** –
   a. Grandiose delusions, e.g. the patient may believe that he is a religious prophet.
   b. Persecutory delusions, e.g. the patient may believe that other people are conspiring against him because of his special importance.
   c. Delusions of reference, e.g. the patient may believe that a remark heard on television is directed specifically to him (i.e. has a personal significance for him).
2. **Hallucinations** –
   a. Usually second person auditory hallucinations – taking the form of voices speaking to the patient about his special powers and consistent with the mood.
   b. A few patients experience visual hallucinations, sometimes with a religious content.

VII. **Cognition** – impaired attention and concentration – patient easily drawn to irrelevances.

VIII. **Insight** – invariably impaired – patient seldom thinks himself ill or in need of treatment.

IX. **Other psychiatric symptoms** – Schneiderian first-rank symptoms of schizophrenia – occur in 10–20% of manic patients.

AETIOLOGY

I. **Genetic** – strong evidence for genetic aetiology provided by:
   1. **Family studies** – prevalence rate in first-degree relatives of patients with bipolar affective disorders is 15–20%. Prevalence rate in first-degree relatives of patients with unipolar affective disorders is 10–15%; cf. prevalence rate in general population of 3–4%.
   2. **Twin studies** –
      a. Bipolar affective disorders – concordance rate in MZ twins is 79%; cf. 19% in DZ twins.
      b. Unipolar affective disorders – concordance rate in MZ twins is 54%; cf. 20% in DZ twins.

II. **Biochemical theories** –
   1. **The monoamine theory of depression** – depressive disorders are due to depletion, and mania to excessive provision, of a monoamine neurotransmitter at one or more sites in the brain. Evidence for this theory:
      a. Reserpine depletes presynaptic vesicles of monoamine stores and can result in depression.
      b. Amphetamines cause the release of monoamines into the synaptic cleft and can result in euphoria.
      c. Monoamine oxidase inhibitors (MAOIs) and monoamine reuptake inhibitors (tricyclic antidepressants) increase the availability of monoamines to postsynaptic receptors and can elevate mood.
      d. Post-mortem studies indicate decreased serotonin turnover in depression.
      e. CSF and urinary studies indicate decreased levels of the breakdown products of noradrenaline and serotonin in some depressed patients.
   2. **Endocrine abnormalities** –
      a. Hypersecretion of cortisol in some depressives.
      b. Decreased thyroid stimulating hormone (TSH) and growth hormone (GH) responses.
   3. **Electrolyte disturbances** –
      a. Intracellular ('residual') sodium increased in depression, further increased in mania.
      b. Changes in erythrocyte membrane sodium–potassium ATPase – active transport of sodium and potassium increases on recovery from mania and depressive disorders.

III. **Psychological theories** –

1. **Maternal deprivation** – deprivation of maternal affection through separation or loss predisposes to depressive disorders in adult life.
2. **Relationships with parents** – patients with mild depressive disorders remember their parents as having been less caring and more over-protective, cf. patients with severe depressive disorders and normal controls.
3. **Psychoanalytic theory** –
   a. **Freud** –
      i. Depression thought to occur when feelings of love and hostility are present at the same time (ambivalence).
      ii. The depressed patient regresses to the oral stage of psychosexual development, at which sadistic feelings are powerful.

   b. **Klein** – if the child does not pass through the 'depressive position' successfully, he will be more likely to develop depression in adult life. The 'depressive position' is the stage of learning where the infant acquires confidence that, when his mother leaves him, she will return even when he has been angry.

   c. **Psychodynamic theory** – mania is a defence against depression.
4. **Cognitive theory** – Beck suggests that a person who habitually adopts ways of thinking with depressive 'cognitive distortions', will be more likely to become depressed when faced with minor problems. There are four basic types of error shown by cognitive distortions in the cognitive theory of depression:
   a. Arbitrary inference – drawing a conclusion when there is no evidence for it and even some against it.
   b. Selective abstraction – focusing on a detail and ignoring more important features of a situation.
   c. Over-generalization – drawing a general conclusion on the basis of a single incident.
   d. Minimization and magnification – performance is underestimated and errors are overestimated.
5. **Learned helplessness** – depression results when highly desirable outcomes are believed improbable or highly aversive outcomes are believed probable, and the individual expects that no response of his will change their likelihood.
6. **Separation experiments in animals** – arise from the suggestion that the loss of a loved person may be a cause of depressive

disorders. The studies may be of some importance to understanding the effects of separating human infants from their mothers.

7. **Premorbid personality** –
   a. Bipolar affective disorders – associated with cyclothymic personality traits (i.e. repeated and sustained mood swings).
   b. Unipolar affective disorders – associated with anankastic personality traits and readiness to develop anxiety.

IV. **Sociological theory** – In Brown's study (1975) of working-class women from inner London boroughs, the vulnerability factors for depression were:
1. Three or more children under 15 years of age at home.
2. Not working outside the home.
3. Lack of a supportive relationship with husband.
4. Loss of mother by death or separation before the age of 11.
5. An excess of threatening life events or major difficulties prior to the onset of depression.

V. **Life event studies** – depressives experience more life events (e.g. bereavement, separation) over normal controls in the six months prior to the onset of the disorder (Paykel, 1969).

VI. **Body build (Kretschmer)** – patients of pyknic (stocky and rounded) build are particularly prone to affective disorders.

DIFFERENTIAL DIAGNOSIS

I. **Depressive disorders** – Exclude:
1. Neuroses.
2. Schizophrenia.
3. Organic disorders – dementia, hypothyroidism.

II. **Mania** – Exclude:
1. Schizophrenia.
2. Organic disorders – frontal lobe tumour, general paralysis of the insane (GPI), drug abuse.

MANAGEMENT

I. **Physical** –

1. **Treatment of depressive disorders** –
   a. **Tricyclic antidepressant drugs** –
      i. Agitated depression – treat with a sedating drug, e.g. amitriptyline.
      ii. Retarded depression – treat with a less sedating drug, e.g. imipramine.
   b. **5-HT reuptake inhibitors** – e.g. fluvoxamine
      i. A highly selective 5-hydroxytryptamine (5-HT) reuptake inhibitor with little or no effect upon noradrenergic processes.
      ii. No daytime sedation in most cases.
      iii. No anticholinergic side-effects.
      iv. No clinically significant cardiovascular side-effects; cf. tricyclic antidepressants.
   c. **Tetracyclic antidepressant drugs** – e.g. mianserin
      i. No anticholinergic side-effects.
      ii. Minimal cardiotoxicity – safer in overdosage.
      iii. Rarely causes convulsions; cf. tricyclic antidepressants.
   d. **Monoamine oxidase inhibitors (MAOIs)** – e.g. phenelzine. Treatment of less severe chronic depressive disorders with prominent anxiety symptoms, which have not responded to a full trial of a cyclic antidepressant drug.
   e. **Lithium carbonate** –
      i. Treatment can be justified in the acute stage of depressive disorders, when other measures have failed.
      ii. Effective in patients who have not responded to a cyclic antidepressant drug.
      iii. Enhances the effects of tricyclic antidepressants and MAOIs.
   f. **Electroconvulsive therapy (ECT)** –
      i. The effects of ECT are best in severe depressive disorders, especially those with marked biological and psychotic features of depression.
      ii. The therapeutic agent is the convulsion.

      N.B. The presence of biological and psychotic features of depression predicts a good response to both ECT and tricyclic antidepressants. Thus, it is mainly the speed of action that distinguishes ECT from tricyclic antidepressant drug treatment (the mood elevating effect with the latter takes two weeks to begin).

2. **Preventing relapse of depressive disorders** –
   a. **Tricyclic antidepressant drugs/5-HT reuptake inhibitors/tetracyclic antidepressant drugs** –
      i. After the first episode of a unipolar affective disorder – if treatment is prolonged for six months after clinical recovery, it reduces the rate of relapse.
      ii. After two or more episodes of a unipolar affective disorder, treatment should be prolonged for twelve months after clinical recovery to reduce the rate of relapse.
   b. **Lithium carbonate** –
      i. In unipolar affective disorders – lithium reduces the rate of relapse. After the first episode – treatment should be prolonged for six months after clinical recovery. After two or more episodes – treatment should be prolonged for twelve months after clinical recovery. Continuing treatment with lithium reduces the rate of relapse after treatment with ECT.
      ii. In bipolar affective disorders – prolonged administration of lithium (five years) prevents relapses into depression.
3. **Treatment of mania** –
   a. **Antipsychotic drugs** – e.g. chlorpromazine, haloperidol
      i. Usually bring the symptoms of acute mania under rapid control.
      ii. Haloperidol is less sedative and causes less postural hypotension, cf. chlorpromazine. Thus, haloperidol is the drug of choice for mania.
      iii. Droperidol is useful in patients who fail to respond to haloperidol (droperidol is a more potent antipsychotic drug than haloperidol).
   b. **Lithium carbonate** – also effective, but the therapeutic response usually only occurs in the second week of treatment. Thus, the response to lithium is slower than the response to antipsychotic drugs.
4. **Preventing relapse of mania** –
   a. **Lithium carbonate** – in bipolar affective disorders – prolonged administration of lithium (five years) prevents relapses into mania.
   b. **Carbamazepine** – in rapid-cycling bipolar affective

disorders, i.e. disorders in which the mood changes rapidly between mania and depression (four or more affective illnesses a year) – carbamazepine is a better prophylactic agent than lithium. Also useful in patients who fail to respond to lithium carbonate.

c. **Sodium valproate** – effective as a mood stabilizer in some manic patients who fail to respond to lithium carbonate and carbamazepine.

d. **Depot antipsychotic medication** – useful in patients who have poor compliance with oral prophylactic medication.

II. **Social** – social manipulation:

1. Rehousing.
2. Family support, e.g. nursery.

III. **Psychological – depressive disorders** –

1. **Psychotherapy** –
   a. **Supportive psychotherapy** –
      i. Part of the management of every depressed patient.
      ii. Intended to sustain patient until other treatments have their effects, or natural recovery occurs.
   b. **Dynamic psychotherapy** –
      i. Some clinicians restrict the use of dynamic psychotherapy to less severe cases.
      ii. Intended to effect change in the patient by – confrontation of defences; clarification; interpretations – new formulations of the problems.
   c. **Interpersonal psychotherapy** – a systematic and standardized treatment approach to relationships and life problems.
   d. **Family therapy** – aims to alleviate the problems that led to the disorder in the identified patient, rather than to achieve some ideal state of a healthy family.
2. **Behaviour therapy** – cognitive behaviour therapy –
   a. As mentioned earlier, Beck suggests that a person who habitually adopts ways of thinking with depressive 'cognitive distortions', will be more likely to become depressed when faced with minor problems.
   b. In cognitive behaviour therapy, the depressive 'cognitive distortions' are identified from present or recent experiences.

c. Patients record such ideas and examine the evidence for and against them.
d. Patients are also encouraged to undertake some of the pleasurable activities that they gave up when they became depressed.
e. In this way, the patients attempt 'cognitive restructuring'.

PROGNOSIS

I. **Bipolar affective disorders** –
1. In these disorders there has been at least one episode of mania, irrespective of whether or not there has been a depressive disorder.
2. Mean age of onset is about thirty years –
   a. But wide variation in age from late teens to late life.
   b. 90% of cases begin before age of fifty (Angst, 1973).
3. Nearly all manic patients recover eventually.
4. Manic illnesses often recur, and subsequent depressive disorder is frequent.
5. The length of remission between episodes of illness becomes shorter up to the third attack, but does not change after that.
6. Personality is well-preserved between episodes of illness.

II. **Unipolar affective disorders** – nearly all young patients recover, though not all elderly patients do so.

CHAPTER 7

Schizophrenia

CLASSIFICATION

I. **Hebephrenic schizophrenia** –
1. Silly and childish behaviour.
2. Prominent affective symptoms and thought disorder.
3. Delusions common but unsystematized.
4. Hallucinations common but non-elaborate.
5. Occurs in adolescents and young adults.

II. **Paranoid schizophrenia** –
1. Prominent well-systematized persecutory or grandiose delusions and hallucinations.
2. Delusional jealousy.
3. Mood and thought processes relatively spared.
4. Patient may appear normal until his abnormal beliefs are uncovered.
5. More common with increasing age.

III. **Simple schizophrenia** –
1. Insidious development of social withdrawal.
2. Odd behaviour and declining performance at work.
3. Absence of delusions, hallucinations and interference with thinking.

IV. **Catatonic schizophrenia** –
1. Stupor; excitement.
2. Waxy flexibility; catalepsy.
3. Echolalia; echopraxia.
4. Automatic obedience; stereotypy.
5. Ambitendence; mannerism.
6. Mitmachen; mitgehen.
7. Negativism; perseveration.

EPIDEMIOLOGY

I. **Age** – median age of onset –
   1. Males – 28 years.
   2. Females – 32 years.

II. **Sex** – equally common among men and women.

III. **Social class** – increased prevalence in lower social classes.

IV. **Season of birth** – increased incidence in winter births.

V. **Birth order** – increased incidence of low birth order if from large family.

VI. **Prevalence rate** – 1% in the general population.

CLINICAL FEATURES

I. **The acute syndrome (positive symptoms)** – main features –
   1. Delusions.
   2. Hallucinations.
   3. Interference with thinking.
   4. Incongruity of affect.
   5. Precipitated by too much social stimulation.

II. **The chronic syndrome (negative symptoms; defect state)** – main features –
   1. Apathy.
   2. Lack of drive and initiative, i.e. diminished volition.
   3. Social withdrawal.
   4. Deterioration of social behaviour, e.g. shouting obscenities in public.
   5. Slowness, i.e. underactivity.
   6. Poverty of speech.
   7. Poverty of thought.
   8. Schizophrenic or formal thought disorder (i.e. loosening of associations).
   9. Blunting of affect.
   10. Age disorientation.
   11. Precipitated by too little social stimulation.

III. **Schneider's first-rank symptoms of schizophrenia** –

1. **Particular forms of auditory hallucination** –
   a. **Third person auditory hallucinations** – two or more voices discussing or aguing about the subject with each other.
   b. **Running commentary** – voices commenting on the subject's actions in the third person.
   c. **Thought echo (audible thoughts)** –
      i. Gedankenlautwerden – the patient experiences a voice speaking his own thoughts as he thinks them.
      ii. Écho de la pensée – the patient experiences a voice repeating his own thoughts immediately after he has thought them.
2. **Interference with thinking** –
   a. **Thought insertion.**
   b. **Thought withdrawal.**
   c. **Thought broadcasting.**
3. **Other symptoms** –
   a. **Primary delusion (delusional perception)** – a false belief which arises fully formed as a sudden intuition, having no discernible connection with any previous interactions or experiences. Frequently preceded by a delusional mood, in which the patient feels something strange and threatening is happening, but is not sure exactly what.
   b. **Somatic hallucinations** – hallucinatory sensations of sexual intercourse attributed to unwanted sexual interference by a persecutor or series of persecutors.
   c. **'Made' volition.**

IV. **Schneider's second-rank symptoms of schizophrenia** –

1. Secondary delusion – a false belief which arises from some preceding morbid experience, e.g. a prevailing mood, an existing delusion or a hallucination.
2. Second person auditory hallucinations (abusive or derogatory) – the patient usually resents such comments; cf. depressive disorders, when the patient accepts them as justified.
3. Visual, tactile, olfactory and gustatory hallucinations.
4. Incongruity or blunting of affect.
5. Formal thought disorder.
6. Catatonic symptoms (disorders of motor activity) – see catatonic schizophrenia.

V. **Other clinical features of schizophrenia** –

1. Neologisms.
2. Metonyms (paraphrasias) – the use of ordinary words in unusual ways.
3. Abnormalities of mood – depression; euphoria; anxiety; irritability.
4. Grandiose delusions.
5. Persecutory delusions.
6. Delusions of reference.
7. Thought blocking.
8. Concrete thinking – difficulty in dealing with abstract ideas.
9. Lack of insight.

AETIOLOGY

I. **Genetic** – strong evidence for genetic aetiology provided by:

1. **Family studies** – the prevalence rates of schizophrenia in relatives of a schizophrenic are as follows:

Relationship to schizophrenic	**Prevalence rate**
Parent of a schizophrenic	5%
Sibling of a schizophrenic	10%
Child of one schizophrenic parent	14%
Child of two schizophrenic parents	46%

Cf. prevalence rate of 1% in the general population.

2. **Twin studies** – concordance rate in MZ twins is 45%; cf. 10% in DZ twins (Gottesmann and Shields, 1972).

3. **Adoption studies** – Heston (1966) studied 47 children whose mothers were schizophrenic, but who were adopted shortly after birth. These children were compared with similarly adopted children, whose mothers were non-schizophrenic. 14% of the group developed schizophrenia; cf. 0% of the controls.

II. **Biochemical theories** –

1. **The dopamine theory of schizophrenia** – schizophrenia results from overactivity of dopamine within the mesolimbic cortical bundle.

a. **Evidence for:**
   i. Amphetamines increase dopamine release and can produce a paranoid psychosis similar to schizophrenia.
   ii. Disulfiram inhibits dopamine-beta-hydroxylase and can exacerbate schizophrenia.
   iii. All effective neuroleptics block dopamine receptors; antipsychotic potency is related to the degree of antidopaminergic activity.
   iv. Monoamine reuptake inhibitors can exacerbate schizophrenia.
   v. Post-mortem studies indicate increased dopamine levels in mesolimbic areas of schizophrenic brains.

b. **Evidence against:**
   i. CSF studies fail to show increased metabolites of dopamine in schizophrenia; i.e. the levels of homovanillic acid (HVA) are reduced.
   ii. Antipsychotics may raise HVA levels.
   iii. Low-dose apomorphine, a dopamine stimulator, can lead to improvement in chronic schizophrenia.
   iv. L-dopa can reduce the negative symptoms of schizophrenia.

2. **The transmethylation theory of schizophrenia** – abnormal methylated metabolites are formed in the brain due to aberrant methylation of monoamines, and produce the psychological symptoms of schizophrenia. This theory is based on the observation that mescaline, a hallucinogen, is an ortho-methylated derivative of dopamine.
   a. **Evidence for**: the methyl donor methionine, when given in conjuction with an MAOI, exacerbates schizophrenic symptoms.
   b. **Evidence against**: the supposed methyl acceptors nicotinamide and nicotinic acid are without therapeutic effect in the treatment of schizophrenia.

III. **Psychological theories** –

1. **Arousal** – some schizophrenics are overaroused. This abnormality is more frequent among the more socially withdrawn chronic patients.
2. **Attention and perception** – schizophrenics cannot concentrate selectively on the important aspects of sensory input. An overwhelming input of stimuli may provide a basis for some of the perceptual abnormalities described by these patients.

3. **Thought disorder** –
   a. **Concrete thinking (Goldstein)** – inability to think in abstract terms; concrete concepts are substituted.
   b. **Over inclusiveness (Cameron)** – inability to conserve conceptual boundaries, with the result that there is an incorporation of irrelevant ideas.
   c. **Personal construct theory (Kelly, Bannister)** – schizophrenics have an abnormally loose personal construct system, which can be measured with the repertory grid. Abnormal constructs might have developed through repeated invalidations of the patient's previous attempts to make sense of the world, perhaps as a result of disordered family communication experienced in childhood.
4. **Psychoanalytic theory** –
   a. **Freud** – schizophrenia is explained in terms of a withdrawal of libido from external objects. Since the withdrawal of libido makes the external world meaningless, the patient attempts to restore meaning by developing abnormal beliefs.
   b. **Klein** – failure to pass through the 'paranoid–schizoid' position adequately, is the basis for the later development of schizophrenia. In the 'paranoid–schizoid' position, the infant is thought to deal with innate aggressive impulses by splitting both his own ego and his representation of his mother into two incompatible parts, one wholly bad and the other wholly good. Only later does the child realize that the same person could be good at one time and bad at another.
   c. **Sullivan** – schizophrenia is explained in terms of interpersonal difficulties.
5. **Premorbid personality** – schizophrenia is associated with schizoid personality traits in a minority of people (see Chapter 3).

IV. **Social processes** –
1. **Farris and Dunham (1939)** – found a raised incidence of schizophrenia in inner-city Chicago. This gave rise to the social causation hypothesis – poverty and deprivation in lower social class areas lead to schizophrenia.
2. **Goldberg and Morrison (1963)** – found that whilst schizophrenics were predominantly found in the lower social classes, they came from families which were distributed evenly throughout all social classes. This gave rise to the social drift

hypothesis – schizophrenia results in the individual's slide down the social scale.

3. **Odegaard (1932)** –
   a. He showed an increased rate of hospital admissions for Norwegian immigrants in the United States, as compared to Norwegians at home, especially due to schizophrenia.
   b. This stimulated debate between:
      i. Social causation – environmental factors associated with migration lead to mental illness.
      ii. Social selection – individuals prone to or suffering from mental illness tend to migrate.
   c. Odegaard favoured social selection for schizophrenia.
4. **Hare (1956)** – schizophrenics often live alone, unmarried, with few friends, i.e. in social isolation.
5. **Clausen and Kohn (1959)** – such social isolation begins before the illness, sometimes in early childhood. Schizophrenics not isolated in early life were not isolated as adults.

V. **Abnormal family processes** –
1. **Disordered family communications** –
   a. **Bateson (1956)** – features of a double-bind:
      i. Occurs when an instruction is given overtly, but contradicted by a second, more covert instruction, i.e. a parent conveys two conflicting and incompatible messages to their child at the same time.
      ii. There is no escape from the situation in which the contradictory instructions are received.
      iii. The double bind leaves the child able to make only ambiguous or meaningless responses.
      iv. When this process persists, this was said to lead to schizophrenia.
   b. **Wynne and Singer (1963)** – suggested that disrupted, non-sequential communications from and between parents, lead to schizophrenia in their child.
2. **Deviant role relationships** –
   a. **Fromm–Reichmann (1948)** –
      i. He suggested the concept of the 'schizophrenogenic' mother, i.e. he found that the mothers of schizophrenics showed an excess of psychological abnormalities; cf. the mothers of neurotic patients and normal controls.

ii. He suggested that these abnormalities might be an important cause of the child's schizophrenia.

b. **Lidz (1957)** – two types of abnormal family pattern:

i. Marital skew – in which one parent yielded to the other's (usually the mother's) eccentricities, which dominated the family.

ii. Marital schism – in which the parents maintained contrary views so that the child has divided loyalties. The inconsistencies, contradictions and lack of role models were said to lead to schizophrenia.

3. **High expressed emotion (Leff and Vaughn)** –

a. Refers to relatives in the patient's family making critical comments, expressing hostility, or showing signs of emotional over-involvement.

b. The relapse rate is highest in patients who are exposed to high expressed emotion ('EE'), have more than thirty five hours per week face to face contact with the key (high 'EE') relative, and are not complying with their antipsychotic medication.

VI. **Neurological abnormalities** –

1. **Non-localizing ('soft') neurological signs** –

a. Astereognosis.

b. Dysgraphaesthesia.

c. Gait abnormalities.

d. Clumsiness.

These abnormalities reflect defects in the integration of proprioceptive and other sensory information.

2. **Thickening of the corpus callosum** – some suggestion of impairment of interhemispheric transfer in schizophrenics.

3. **Ventricular enlargement** –

a. Widening of sulci, atrophy of cerebellar vermis.

b. Some evidence that patients with ventricular enlargement have more negative symptoms of schizophrenia.

c. Some evidence that such patients perform poorly on tests of intellectual function.

4. **Changes in the EEG** –

a. Increased theta activity.

b. Fast activity.

c. Paroxysmal activity.

5. **Virus-like material** – isolated from the CSF of schizophrenics. Virus infection may be a major cause of schizophrenia.

VII. **Life event studies** – schizophrenics experience more life events over normal controls in the three weeks prior to the onset of acute symptoms of schizophrenia (Brown and Birley, 1968).

VIII. **Body build (Kretschmer)** – patients of asthenic (lean and narrow) build are particularly prone to schizophrenia.

DIAGNOSIS

I. Definite evidence of Schneiderian first-rank symptoms – indicates a diagnosis of schizophrenia, provided that there is no evidence of an organic disorder.

II. In the absence of Schneiderian first-rank symptoms – a diagnosis of schizophrenia can still be made if there is evidence of a prolonged course together with definite evidence of the negative symptoms of schizophrenia.

DIFFERENTIAL DIAGNOSIS

I. **Exclude organic disorders** –
   1. **Among younger patients** –
      a. Drug-induced psychosis –
         i. Amphetamine abuse.
         ii. Alcohol abuse.
      b. Temporal lobe epilepsy (complex partial seizures).
   2. **Among older patients** –
      a. Acute organic syndrome – e.g. encephalitis.
      b. Dementia.
      c. Diffuse brain diseases – e.g. general paralysis of the insane (GPI).
   3. **In addition** – a schizophrenic syndrome can occur post partum and in the post-operative period.

II. **Exclude affective disorders.**

III. **Exclude personality disorders.**

MANAGEMENT

I. **Physical** –

1. **Antipsychotic drugs** –
    a. **Treatment of acute schizophrenia** –
        i. Drug treatment has most effect on the positive symptoms of schizophrenia, and least effect on the negative symptoms of schizophrenia.
        ii. The various antipsychotic drugs do not differ in therapeutic effectiveness, although their side-effects vary.
        iii. The maximum recommended daily dose of chlorpromazine is 1 g (i.e. 250 mg q.d.s.).
        iv. The maximum recommended daily dose of haloperidol is 200 mg (i.e. 50 mg q.d.s.).
        v. Chlorpromazine is more sedative and causes less extrapyramidal side-effects (EPSE), cf. haloperidol; thus, chlorpromazine is the drug of choice for schizophrenia.

    b. **Treatment after the acute phase** –
        i. There is a widespread clinical impression that, in preventing relapses of schizophrenia, depot injections are more successful than continued oral medication.
        ii. In the long-term management of schizophrenia, there is no difference in the usefulness of the various antipsychotic depot injections available. Moreover, the incidence of EPSE is similar for all the depot injections.
        iii. The depot injection should be given indefinitely.
        iv. The maximum recommended dose of fluphenazine decanoate (Modecate) is 100 mg repeated at intervals of fourteen days.
        v. In patients who fail to respond to chlorpromazine and depot antipsychotic medication, a trial of clozepine tablets is worthwhile, providing such patients are monitored closely with regular blood tests to detect any possible agranulocytosis (life-threatening side-effect of clozepine).

2. **ECT** – the traditional indications for ECT in the treatment of schizophrenia are:
    a. The stupor or excitement of catatonic schizophrenia.
    b. Severe depressive symptoms accompanying schizophrenia.

II. **Social** –
1. **Work with relatives** – counselling should be beneficial to families, especially when directed at reducing their expressed emotion; the patient may need to be separated from this.
2. **Rehabilitation of the patient** – using: day hospitals; half-way houses; sheltered workshops. Understimulation or overstimulation of the patient should be avoided.

III. **Psychological** –
1. **Psychotherapy** – supportive psychotherapy, counselling and advice to the patient are always required.
2. **Behaviour therapy** –
    a. **Social skills training** –
        i. Procedure applied to patients with social deficits consequent upon schizophrenia.
        ii. Video recordings are used to define and rate elements of the patient's behaviour in standard social encounters.
        iii. The patient is then taught more appropriate behaviour by a combination of direct instruction, modelling, video-feedback and role reversal.
    b. **Token economy** –
        i. Useful for institutionalized chronic schizophrenics.
        ii. This system uses positive and negative reinforcement to alter behaviour; it is usual to give tokens that can be used to purchase goods or privileges.

PROGNOSIS

I. **'The rule of quarters'** –
1. 25% – remit completely after a first attack of schizophrenia with no further symptoms.
2. 25% – show good social recovery but with some persistence of symptoms.
3. 25% – show partial social recovery with persistence of symptoms.
4. 25% – follow a steadily downhill course with social deterioration, personality deterioration, and in some cases, ending with the defect state.

II. **Good prognostic features** –

1. Acute onset.
2. Presence of a precipitating factor.
3. Prominence of affective symptoms.
4. Older age at onset.
5. Short episode.
6. No past psychiatric history.
7. Good premorbid personality.
8. Good psychosexual adjustment.
9. Good social relationships.
10. Good work record.
11. Married.

III. **Causes of relapse** –

1. Iatrogenic relapse i.e. the doctor reducing the patient's medication in an attempt to minimize the risk of tardive dyskinesia – commonest cause of relapse.
2. Non-compliance with medication – second commonest cause of relapse
3. High 'EE' – third commonest cause of relapse.

CHAPTER 8

Organic Disorders

CLASSIFICATION

I. **Acute organic disorder (delirium)** –
   1. Acute onset.
   2. Fluctuating course.

II. **Chronic organic disorder (dementia)** –
   1. Insidious onset.
   2. Steady progressive course.

CLINICAL FEATURES

I. **Acute organic disorder** –
   1. **Consciousness** – impairment of consciousness recognized by:
      a. Slowness.
      b. Uncertainty about the time of day.
      c. Poor concentration.
   2. **Behaviour** – two possible forms –
      a. Overactivity, noisiness, repetitive purposeless movements.
      b. Inactivity, slowness, repetitive purposeless movements.
   3. **Speech** – reduced speech.
   4. **Mood** –
      a. Anxiety.
      b. Irritability.
      c. Depression.
      d. Lability of mood.
      e. Perpelexed or frightened and agitated.
   5. **Thought** –
      a. Slow and muddled – but often rich in content.
      b. Ideas of reference and persecutory delusions – transient and poorly elaborated.
      c. Perseveration.

6. **Perception** –
   a. Visual illusions, visual misinterpretations and visual hallucinations – may have a fantastic content.
   b. Tactile and auditory hallucinations.
   c. Depersonalization and derealization.
7. **Cognition** –
   a. Disorientation in time and place.
   b. Disturbance of memory – affecting registration, retention, recall and new learning.
8. **Insight** – impaired.

II. **Chronic organic disorder** –
1. **Consciousness** – no impairment of consciousness (i.e. clear consciousness). Global impairment of cerebral functions – i.e. generalized impairment of intellect, personality and memory.
2. **Behaviour** –
   a. Shrinkage of the milieu – reduction of interests.
   b. Organic orderliness – rigid and stereotyped routines.
   c. Catastrophic reaction – when the person is taxed beyond restricted abilities, there is a sudden explosion of anger or other emotion.
3. **Speech** –
   a. Syntactical errors and nominal dysphasia.
   b. Eventually patient may utter only meaningless noises or become mute.
4. **Mood** –
   a. Anxiety.
   b. Irritability.
   c. Depression.
   d. Lability of mood.
5. **Thought** –
   a. Slow and impoverished in content.
   b. Persecutory delusions.
   c. Perseveration.
   d. Concrete thinking.
6. **Perception** – hallucinations.
7. **Cognition** –
   a. Disorientation in time, place and person.
   b. Impaired attention and concentration.
   c. Disturbance of memory –
      i. Forgetfulness.

  - ii. Difficulty in new learning is generally the most conspicuous sign.
  - iii. Memory loss is more obvious for recent than for remote events.
  - iv. Patients may use confabulation to hide memory deficits, i.e. apparent recollection of imaginary events and experiences.

8. **Insight** – impaired.

AETIOLOGY

I. **Acute organic disorder** –
  1. **Alcohol/drugs** –
     - a. Alcohol or other drug intoxication (e.g. L-dopa, anticholinergics, anxiolytic–hypnotics, anticonvulsants, opiates).
     - b. Withdrawal of alcohol or other drugs.
  2. **Metabolic causes** –
     - a. Uraemia.
     - b. Electrolyte imbalance (e.g. hypercalcaemia).
     - c. Cardiac failure.
     - d. Respiratory failure.
     - e. Hepatic failure.
     - f. Acute intermittent porphyria.
     - g. Systemic lupus erythematosus (SLE).
  3. **Endocrine causes** –
     - a. Hyperthyroidism.
     - b. Hypothyroidism.
     - c. Hypoparathyroidism.
     - d. Hypopituitarism.
     - e. Hypoglycaemia.
  4. **Infective causes** –
     - a. **Intercranial infection** –
       - i. Encephalitis.
       - ii. Meningitis.
     - b. **Systemic infection** –
       - i. Septicaemia.
       - ii. Pneumonia.
  5. **Other intracranial causes** –
     - a. Space-occupying lesion.
     - b. Raised intracranial pressure.

6. **Vitamin deficiency** –
   a. B_1 (thiamine) – Wernicke's encephalopathy.
   b. B_{12}.
   c. Nicotinic acid.
7. **Head injury.**
8. **Heavy metals** – heavy metal intoxication (e.g. lead, manganese).
9. **Epilepsy.**

II. **Chronic organic disorder** –
1. **Degenerative causes** –
   a. Senile dementia of the Alzheimer type (SDAT).
   b. Alzheimer's disease.
   c. Multi-infarct dementia (MID).
   d. Pick's disease.
   e. Parkinson's disease.
   f. Huntington's chorea.
   g. Normal pressure hydrocephalus (communicating hydrocephalus).
   h. Multiple sclerosis (disseminated sclerosis).
   i. Jakob–Creutzfeld's disease (JCD).
   j. Subacute spongiform encephalopathy.
   k. Subcortical dementia.
   l. Punch drunk syndrome.
2. **Metabolic causes** –
   a. Sustained uraemia.
   b. Electrolyte imbalance (e.g. hypocalcaemia).
   c. Chronic respiratory failure.
   d. Chronic hepatic failure.
   e. Chronic renal failure.
   f. Wilson's disease.
   g. SLE.
3. **Endocrine causes** – hypothyroidism.
4. **Infective causes** – intracranial infection –
   a. Encephalitis.
   b. Neurosyphilis – general paralysis of the insane (GPI).
   c. Cerebral sarcoidosis.
5. **Other intracranial causes** – space-occupying lesion (e.g. tumour, subdural haematoma).
6. **Vitamin deficiency** – sustained lack of:
   a. B_1 – Korsakoff's psychosis.
   b. B_{12} – subacute combined degeneration of the cord.
   c. Nicotinic acid – pellagra.

7. **Head injury.**
8. **Alcohol/heavy metals** – alcohol or heavy metal intoxication (e.g. lead, arsenic, thallium).
9. **Anoxia** –
   a. Cardiac arrest.
   b. Carbon monoxide poisoning.
   c. Anaemia.
   d. Post-anaesthesia.

DIAGNOSIS

I. **Senile dementia of the Alzheimer type** –
   1. **Memory failure.**
   2. **Lability of mood.**
   3. **Apathy.**
   4. **Depressive or paranoid features.**
   5. **Parkinsonism.**
   6. **Parietal lobe syndrome** –
      a. Constructional apraxia – the inability to copy two-dimensional drawings or to construct three-dimensional models.
      b. Dressing apraxia – the inability to put clothing on properly.
      c. Ideational apraxia – the inability to voluntarily carry out a sequence of actions.
      d. Ideomotor apraxia – the inability to copy gestures.
      e. Anosognosia – denial of the disorder.
      f. Topographical agnosia – getting lost in familiar surroundings.
      g. Hemisomatognosia – neglecting one side of the body.
      h. Autotopagnosia – the inability to recognize, name, or point on command to parts of the body.
      i. Sensory inattention.
      j. Cortical sensory loss.
      k. Astereognosis – the inability to identify objects when placed in the hand.
      l. Epilepsy.
      m. Aspects of Gerstmann's syndrome (seen in dominant lobe lesions) –
         i. Right–left disorientation.
         ii. Finger agnosia – the inability to name fingers.
         iii. Dyscalculia – difficulty with calculations.

iv. Dysgraphia – difficulty in expressing ideas in writing.

7. **Mirror sign** – the inability to identify one's own image.
8. **Logoclonia** – the monotonous repetition of word particles.
9. **Epilepsy.**
10. **Relentless progress of personality and intellectual deterioration.**
11. **Aspects of the Kluver–Bucy syndrome** –
    a. Hyperorality.
    b. Hypersexuality.
    c. Increased need to touch.
    d. Placidity.
    e. Visual agnosia.
    f. Defects in language and in memory.

II. **Alzheimer's disease** – the same disorder as senile dementia of the Alzheimer type, except that it is pre-senile.

III. **Multi-infarct dementia** –
1. Stepwise deterioration in memory.
2. Perseveration.
3. Fluctuating cognitive impairment.
4. Episodes of nocturnal confusion.
5. Depression.
6. Hypertension.
7. Headache.
8. Dizziness.
9. Tinnitus.
10. Scotomata.
11. Apraxias – the inability to perform voluntary motor acts.
12. Agnosias – the inability to understand the significance of sensory stimuli.
13. Aphasia.
14. Focal neurological deficits.
15. Personality preservation until late.
16. Insight intact.

IV. **Pick's disease** –
1. **Frontal lobe syndrome** :
    a. Disinhibition.
    b. Facetious humour, euphoria.
    c. Irritability, apathy.
    d. Loss of initiative, decreased intellectual drive.
    e. Loss of ethical standards, expressive dysphasia.

f. Grasp reflex, urinary incontinence.
g. Tactlessness, overtalkativeness.
h. Reduced verbal fluency, reduced fine motor control.
i. Excess in drinking and eating, excess in sexual behaviour.
j. Gegenhalten, contralateral spastic paresis.
k. Impaired spelling, difficulty in programming and planning behaviour.

2. **Personality deterioration.**
3. **Nominal aphasia.**
4. **Perseveration.**
5. **Amnesia.**
6. **Generalized hyperalgesia.**

V. **Huntington's chorea** –

1. Insidious onset of choreo-athetoid movements.
2. Slurring of speech.
3. Ataxic gait.
4. Intention tremor.
5. Rigidity.
6. Epilepsy.
7. Apathy.
8. Depression.
9. Irritability.
10. Distractibility.
11. Insidious onset of global dementia.
12. Paranoid state.

DIFFERENTIAL DIAGNOSIS

I. **Exclude functional psychiatric disorders** –

1. Affective disorders.
2. Schizophrenia.

II. **Differentiate dementia from depressive pseudodementia** –
Distinguishing features of depressive pseudodementia –

1. Conspicuous subjective difficulty in concentration and remembering but careful clinical testing shows there is no defect of memory function.
2. Psychological symptoms precede the apparent intellectual defects – hence it is important to interview other informants to determine the precise mode of onset.

3. Relatively acute onset.
4. Absence of focal signs.
5. Abreaction or sleep deprivation may clarify the diagnosis.

III. **Differentiate dementia from hysterical pseudodementia (including Ganser's syndrome)** –
Features of Ganser's syndrome –
1. The giving of approximate answers, i.e. answers to simple questions that are plainly wrong but strongly suggest that the correct answer is known.
2. Apparent clouding of consciousness.
3. Hysterical dissociative symptoms, e.g. psychogenic amnesia.
4. Hysterical conversion symptoms, e.g. ataxia.
5. Pseudohallucinations.

MANAGEMENT

I. **Acute organic disorder** –
1. **Specific measures** –
    a. The fundamental treatment is directed to the physical cause.
    b. In some cases – the effect of appropriate treatment is quite immediate and dramatic, and little more treatment is required, e.g. in the case of hypoglycaemia.
    c. In most cases – recovery is more protracted and it is important to observe certain general measures.
2. **General measures** –
    a. The patient should be nursed in a well-lit room, preferably a side ward.
    b. Medical and nursing staff should reassure the patient, and explain to him both where he is and what is the purpose of any examination or treatment.
    c. The patient should be comfortable, adequately hydrated and in electrolyte balance.
3. **Drug treatment** –
    a. **During the daytime** –
        i. It may be necessary to calm the patient without inducing drowsiness.
        ii. The drug choice is haloperidol, which calms without causing drowsiness and postural hypotension, cf. chlorpromazine.

  - iii. The effective daily dose of haloperidol usually varies from 10 to 60 mg.
- b. **At night** –
  - i. It may be necessary to help the patient sleep.
  - ii. A suitable drug is a sedative anxiolytic drug (i.e. a benzodiazepine) which promotes sleep.
- c. **In the special case of alcohol withdrawal** – chlormethiazole is a suitable drug.
- d. **In the special case of hepatic failure** – benzodiazepines may be used during the daytime despite their sedative effects, since they are less likely to precipitate coma, cf. haloperidol.

II. **Chronic organic disorder** –

1. **Specific measures** –
   - a. If possible the cause should be treated.
   - b. It is important to detect those cases where treatment can have a marked benefit; for example –
     - i. Normal pressure hydrocephalus.
     - ii. Hypocalcaemia.
     - iii. Chronic renal failure.
     - iv. Wilson's disease.
     - v. Hypothyroidism.
     - vi. GPI.
     - vii. Space-occupying lesion.
     - viii. Vitamin B_{12} deficiency.
     - ix. Alcohol or heavy metal intoxication.
2. **General measures** –
   - a. The most important consideration – adequate help with self care and prevention of accidental self harm.
   - b. Most early cases and many advanced cases – can be managed at home with suitable support, e.g. home helps, district nurses.
3. **Drug treatment** –
   - a. There is no specific drug treatment for dementia.
   - b. Medication can only be used to alleviate certain symptoms –
     - i. **Anxiety** – treated with a benzodiazepine or a phenothiazine (e.g. thioridazine, chlorpromazine).
     - ii. **Depressive symptoms** – a trial of antidepressant medication is worthwhile even in the presence of dementia.

iii. **Overactivity/delusions/hallucinations** – a phenothiazine may be appropriate, but care is needed to find the optimal dose.

iv. **Cognitive impairment** – patients with this may be unusually sensitive to antipsychotic drugs; thus, the first doses should be small.

CHAPTER 9

Eating Disorders

ANOREXIA NERVOSA

Definition

An extreme exaggeration of the widespread habit of dieting. Generally begins with ordinary efforts at dieting in a girl who is somewhat overweight at the time.

Epidemiology

I. **Age** –
   1. **Females** –
      a. Onset usually between ages 16–17.
      b. Onset seldom after the age of 30.
   2. **Males** – onset usually about the age of 12.

II. **Sex** –
   1. More common in females.
   2. The ratio of females to males is about 10:1.

III. **Social class** – more common in upper social classes, i.e. social classes I and II.

IV. **Prevalence rate** – 1% of middle-class adolescent girls.

V. **Incidence** – increasing incidence in recent years – probably due to social pressures.

Clinical features

I. **Main clinical features** –
   1. A body weight more than 25% below the standard weight.
   2. An intense wish to be thin.
   3. Amenorrhoea (in women).

II. **Central psychological features** –
   1. A fear of being fat.

2. Relentless pursuit of a low body weight.
3. The patient has a distorted image of her body – believing herself to be too fat even when severely underweight.

III. **The pursuit of thinness** – this may take several forms:
1. Patients generally eat very little and show a particular avoidance of carbohydrates.
2. Some patients try to achieve this by inducing vomiting, excessive exercise and purging.
3. Some patients have episodes of uncontrollable overeating (binge eating or bulimia):
    a. After overeating, they feel bloated and may induce vomiting.
    b. Binges are followed by remorse and intensified efforts to lose weight.

IV. **Physical consequences** –
1. **Clinical features secondary to starvation** –
    a. Sensitivity to cold.
    b. Constipation.
    c. Low blood pressure.
    d. Bradycardia.
    e. Hypothermia.
    f. Amenorrhoea (also a primary symptom in a few cases – see earlier).
    g. Leucopenia.
    h. Abnormalities of water regulation.
2. **Consequences of vomiting and laxative abuse** –
    a. Hypokalaemia.
    b. Alkalosis.
    c. Epilepsy.
    d. Cardiac arrhythmia.
3. **Hormonal abnormalities** –
    a. Elevated hormone levels –
        i. Growth hormone (GH).
        ii. Prolactin.
        iii. Cortisol.
    b. Reduced hormone levels –
        i. Tri-iodothyronine (T_3).
        ii. Thyroxine (T_4).
        iii. Oestradiol.
        iv. Testosterone.

v. Follicle-stimulating hormone (FSH).
vi. Luteinizing hormone (LH).

Aetiology

I. **Genetic** – 6–10% of female siblings of patients with established anorexia nervosa suffer with the condition.

II. **Hypothalamic dysfunction** – with abnormal control of food intake and reduced sex hormones, which show delayed return on recovery of normal weight.

III. **Social factors** –
1. High prevalence in upper and middle social classes.
2. High prevalence in occupational groups particularly concerned with weight, e.g. ballet students.

IV. **Individual psychological causes** –
1. **Disturbance of body image** – the three predisposing factors are:
    a. Dietary problems in early life.
    b. Parents who are preoccupied with food.
    c. Family relationships that leave the child without a sense of identity.
2. **Analytical model** –
    a. Regression to childhood.
    b. Fixation at oral (pregenital) level of psychosexual development.
    c. Escape from the emotional problems of adolescence.

V. **Causes within the family** –
1. A specific pattern of relationships can be identified – consisting of:
    a. Enmeshment.
    b. Overprotectiveness.
    c. Rigidity.
    d. Lack of conflict resolution.
2. Development of anorexia nervosa in patient serves to prevent dissension within the family.

Differential diagnosis

I. **Exclude functional psychiatric illnesses** –
1. Phobic anxiety neuroses.
2. Obsessive compulsive neuroses.

3. Depressive disorders.
4. Schizophrenia.

II. **Exclude organic disorders** –
1. Hypopituitarism.
2. Thyrotoxicosis.
3. Malabsorption.
4. Diabetes mellitus.
5. Neoplasia.
6. Reticuloses.

Management

I. **Physical** – chlorpromazine and tricyclic antidepressants may be used to promote weight gain. However, the effect is temporary and drug treatment has been superseded by psychological treatment in most centres.

II. **Social** – successful treatment largely depends on making a good relationship with the patient, so that a firm approach is possible. It should be made clear that the maintenance of an adequate weight is an essential first priority.

III. **Psychological** –
1. **Psychotherapy** –
   a. **Supportive psychotherapy** – directed to improving personal relationships and increasing the patient's sense of personal effectiveness.
   b. **Family therapy** – has been advocated since problems in family relationships are common in anorexia nervosa.
2. **Behaviour therapy** –
   a. **Carefully controlled calorie intake** –
      i. A strict regime of refeeding is carried out.
      ii. Usually behavioural principles are used – i.e. a target weight is set and the patient gains privileges by increasing her weight; e.g. having visitors, trips out of her room.
      iii. Carried out as an in-patient.
   b. **Cognitive behaviour therapy** –
      i. Aimed at changing the patient's attitude towards eating, and reappraisal of her self-image and life circumstances.
      ii. Usually carried out as an out-patient.

Prognosis

I. **Untreated cases** – the prognosis is very poor.

II. **Treated cases** – the rule of thirds –
1. One third – recover fully.
2. One third – recover somewhat.
3. One third – little improved or chronically disabled.

III. **Factors associated with a poor prognosis** –
1. Long illness.
2. Late age of onset.
3. Bulimia.
4. Vomiting or purging.
5. Anxiety when eating in the presence of others.
6. Great weight loss.
7. Poor childhood social adjustment.
8. Poor parental relationships.
9. Male sex.

IV. **Mortality rate** – 5–10%.

CHAPTER 10

Alcohol/Drug Dependence

ALCOHOL DEPENDENCE

Definition

The seven essential elements in the alcohol dependence syndrome are:

I. Subjective awareness of compulsion to drink.
II. Stereotyped pattern of drinking.
III. Increased tolerance to alcohol.
IV. Primacy of drinking over other activities.
V. Repeated withdrawal symptoms.
VI. Relief drinking.
VII. Reinstatement after abstinence.

Epidemiology

I. **Age** –
  1. Heaviest drinkers – men in their late teens or early twenties.
  2. Increasing incidence among adolescents.

II. **Sex** –
  1. More common in males.
  2. Increasing incidence among females.

III. **Social class** – lowest prevalence in middle social classes.

IV. **Marital status** – more common in divorced or separated.

V. **Occupation** – certain high-risk occupations, e.g. company directors, doctors.

VI. **Ethnic factors** –
  1. More common in Irish people.
  2. Less common in Jewish people.

Clinical features (psychiatric aspects)

Alcohol-related psychiatric disorders – four groups –

I. **Intoxication phenomena** –
   1. **Pathological drunkenness** – acute psychotic episodes induced by relatively small amounts of alcohol –
      a. Individual idiosyncratic reactions to alcohol.
      b. Usually take the form of explosive outbursts of aggression.
   2. **Memory blackouts** – short-term amnesia –
      a. Fragmentary lapses to several hours.
      b. Frequently reported after heavy drinking.

II. **Withdrawal phenomena** –
   1. **General withdrawal symptoms** –
      a. Acute tremulousness affecting the hands, legs and trunk ('the shakes').
      b. Agitation.
      c. Nausea.
      d. Retching.
      e. Sweating.
      f. Perceptual distortions and hallucinations.
      g. Convulsions.
   2. **Delirium tremens** – the fully developed withdrawal syndrome –
      a. Clouding of consciousness.
      b. Disorientation in time and place.
      c. Impairment of recent memory.
      d. Illusions.
      e. Hallucinations.
      f. Delusions.
      g. Agitation and restlessness.
      h. Fearful affect.
      i. Prolonged insomnia.
      j. Tremulous hands.
      k. Truncal ataxia.
      l. Autonomic overactivity.

III. **Nutritional or toxic disorders** –
   1. **Sustained lack of thiamine** –
      a. **Wernicke's encephalopathy** –
         i. Ophthalmoplegia.
         ii. Nystagmus.
         iii. Clouding of consciousness with memory disturbance.
         iv. Ataxia.
         v. Peripheral neuropathy.

b. **Korsakoff's psychosis** –
   i. Impairment of recent memory.
   ii. Confabulation.
   iii. Retrograde amnesia.
   iv. Disorientation.
   v. Euphoria.
   vi. Apathy.
   vii. Lack of insight.
   viii. Ataxia.
   ix. Peripheral neuropathy.

2. **Alcoholic dementia.**

IV. **Associated psychiatric disorders** –
   1. **Alcoholic hallucinosis** –
      a. Auditory hallucinations occurring alone in clear consciousness.
      b. Voices usually utter insults or threats; may be followed by secondary delusional interpretation.
      c. The patient is usually distressed by these experiences, appearing anxious and restless.
   2. **Affective disorder.**
   3. **Personality deterioration.**
   4. **Suicidal behaviour.**
   5. **Sexual problems.**
   6. **Pathological jealousy** – the delusion that the marital partner is being unfaithful.

Aetiology

I. **Genetic factors** –
   1. **Twin studies** – show higher concordance rates in MZ than DZ twins.
   2. **Adoption study** – Goodwin (1973) showed significantly higher levels of alcoholism in individuals whose biological parents were known alcoholics and who were adopted in childhood, than in a matched control group.

II. **Biochemical factors** – abnormalities in:
   1. Alcohol dehydrogenase.
   2. Neurotransmitter mechanisms.

III. **Learning factors** – children tend to follow their parents' drinking patterns.

IV. **Personality factors** – alcohol dependence associated with:
1. Chronic anxiety.
2. Self-indulgent tendencies.
3. A pervading sense of inferiority.

V. **Psychiatric illness** – alcohol dependence occurs in patients with:
1. Anxiety neuroses.
2. Phobic anxiety neuroses.
3. Affective disorders.
4. Schizophrenia.
5. Organic disorders.

VI. **Alcohol consumption in society** – rate of alcohol dependence is related to the general level of alcohol consumption in society.

Management

I. **Physical** – detoxification, i.e. the management of withdrawal of alcohol –
1. **Sedation** –
   a. Chlormethiazole (Heminevrin) or chlordiazepoxide (Librium) – sedative drugs generally prescribed to reduce withdrawal symptoms.
   b. Chlormethiazole may be prescribed in either of 2 ways:
      i. On an as-required basis – i.e. flexibly according to the patient's symptoms.
      ii. On a reducing regime basis – i.e. on a fixed 6-hourly regime of gradually decreasing dosage over 6–9 days.
   c. The patient must stop drinking when taking chlormethiazole – if chlormethiazole is taken in combination with alcohol, each potentiates the CNS depressant action of the other, and overdosage is frequently fatal.
2. **Vitamin supplements** – to provide thiamine: two possible forms –
   a. Intramuscular or intravenous injections of parentrovite for 5 days.
   b. Oral multivitamin tablets which contain thiamine.
3. **Rehydration** – to correct any electrolyte imbalance.
4. **Glucose** – to correct any hypoglycaemia.
5. **Antibiotics** – to treat any infection.
6. **Anticonvulsants** – to treat any convulsions, e.g. large doses of chlordiazepoxide may be used.

II. **Social** –

1. **A goal-orientated treatment plan** – these goals should deal with:
    a. **The drinking problem** –
        i. Total abstinence – a better goal for those aged over 40, who are heavily dependent on alcohol and have incurred physical damage, and who have attempted controlled drinking unsuccessfully.
        ii. Controlled drinking – a feasible goal for those under 40, who are not heavily dependent on alcohol and have not incurred physical damage, and whose problem has been detected early.
    b. **Any accompanying problems in** –
        i. Health.
        ii. Marriage.
        iii. Job.
        iv. Social adjustment.
2. **Other agencies concerned with drinking problems** –
    a. **Alcoholics Anonymous (AA)** –
        i. The meetings involve an emotional confession of problems.
        ii. Any patient aiming for abstinence should be recommended to try this organization.
    b. **Hostels** –
        i. Provide rehabilitation and counselling; usually abstinence is a condition of residence.
        ii. Intended mainly for homeless problem drinkers.

III. **Psychological** –

1. **Psychotherapy** –
    a. **Supportive psychotherapy** – simple counselling and advice –
        i. To educate the patient about the physical, social and psychological complications of alcohol dependence.
        ii. To help the patient cope with problems in day-to-day living without drinking to excess.
    b. **Group psychotherapy** –
        i. Aims to enable patients to:
            – Observe their own problems mirrored in other problem drinkers.
            – Work out better ways of coping with their problems.
        ii. The most widely used treatment for problem drinkers.

2. **Behaviour therapy** –
   a. Tackles the drinking behaviour itself rather than the underlying psychological problems.
   b. Includes simple approaches such as self-monitoring, e.g. getting the patient to keep a strict daily log of drinking.
   c. Often effective.

Prognosis

Factors predicting a good prognosis –

1. First treatment.
2. Motivated.
3. Social stability – in form of:
   a. A fixed abode.
   b. Family support.
   c. Ability to keep a job.
4. Absence of antisocial personality traits – i.e. the ability to:
   a. Control impulsiveness.
   b. Defer gratification.
   c. Form deep emotional relationships.
5. Older.
6. Adequate intelligence.
7. Good insight into nature of the problems.

DRUG DEPENDENCE

Definition

A state, psychic and sometimes also physical, resulting from the interaction between a living organism and a drug, characterized by behavioural and other responses that always include a compulsion to take the drug on a continuous or periodic basis in order to experience its psychic effects and sometimes to avoid the discomfort of its absence.

Tolerance may or may not be present.

Epidemiology

I. **Age** –
   1. Most common in age group 20–30s.
   2. Slight peak in middle age.

II. **Sex** – More common among males.

III. **Social class** –
  1. **UK** – occurs throughout all social classes.
  2. **USA** – associated with underprivileged, minority, ethnic groups.

Clinical features

I. **Opiates** – e.g. heroin.
  1. Both psychic and physical dependence occur.
  2. **Clinical features of chronic opiate dependence** –
     a. Constipation.
     b. Constricted pupils.
     c. Chronic malaise.
     d. Weakness.
     e. Impotence.
     f. Tremors.
  3. **Withdrawal effects from opiates** –
     a. Pilo-erection; shivering.
     b. Abdominal cramps; diarrhoea.
     c. Lacrimation; rhinorrhoea.
     d. Dilated pupils; tachycardia.
     e. Yawning; intense craving for drug.
     f. Agitation; restlessness.

II. **Barbiturates** – e.g. pentobarbitone.
  1. Both psychic and physical dependence occur.
  2. **Clinical features of barbiturate dependence** –
     a. Slurred speech.
     b. Incoherence.
     c. Dullness.
     d. Drowsiness.
     e. Nystagmus.
     f. Depression.
  3. **Withdrawal effects from barbiturates** –
     a. Clouding of consciousness; disorientation.
     b. Hallucinations; major seizures.
     c. Anxiety and restlessness.
     d. Pyrexia and tremulousness.
     e. Insomnia and hypotension.
     f. Nausea; vomiting.
     g. Anorexia; twitching.

III. **Hallucinogens** – e.g. lysergic acid diethylamide (LSD).
  1. Psychic dependence occurs. Physical dependence does not occur.

2. **The mental effects of LSD**:
   a. Develop during the two hours after LSD consumption; usually last from 8 to 14 hours.
   b. Unpredictable and extremely dangerous behaviour; the user sometimes injuring or killing himself through behaving as if he were invulnerable.
   c. Mood – acute anxiety, distress or exhilaration.
   d. Distortions or intensifications of sensory perception –
      i. Synaesthesia – confusion between sensory modalities, e.g. movements are experienced as if heard.
      ii. Distortion of the body image – the person sometimes feels that he is outside his own body.

   These experiences may lead to panic with fears of insanity.

IV. **Amphetamines** – e.g. dexamphetamine.
1. Psychic dependence occurs. Physical dependence does not occur.
2. **Amphetamine psychosis** –
   a. Excessive or chronic use of amphetamines, whether taken by mouth or intravenously, induces a paranoid psychosis indistinguishable from acute paranoid schizophrenia.
   b. **Features** –
      i. Hostile and dangerously aggressive behaviour.
      ii. Prominent persecutory delusions.
      iii. Auditory, visual and tactile hallucinations.
      iv. Clear consciousness.
   c. The condition usually subsides on discontinuing the drug over about a week; however, a few cases continue for months.
   d. It is uncertain whether amphetamine psychosis is a case of schizophrenia provoked by amphetamines, or a true drug-induced psychosis.

V. **Cannabis** – active principle is tetrahydro-cannabinol.
1. Psychic dependence occurs. Physical dependence does not occur.
2. **The effects of cannabis** –
   a. Exaggerates the pre-existing mood – whether euphoria, depression or anxiety.
   b. Distortion of time and space.
   c. Increased enjoyment of aesthetic experiences.
   d. Intensification of visual perception and visual hallucinations.
   e. Dry mouth; coughing.
   f. Increased appetite; decreased body temperature.

g. Reddening of the eyes; irritation of the respiratory tract.

3. **The adverse effects of cannabis** –
   a. A chronic 'amotivation syndrome' in heavy users – blunted motivation, i.e. apathy, decreased drive, lack of ambition.
   b. Psychotic reactions – in patients with a pre-existing psychosis or a vulnerability to psychosis.
   c. Transient 'flashback' phenomena.

VI. **Cocaine** –
1. Psychic dependence occurs. Physical dependence does not occur.
2. **Formication ('cocaine bugs')** –
   a. Characteristic of cocaine dependence.
   b. A bizarre tactile hallucination in which there is a feeling as though insects are crawling under the skin.

VII. **Benzodiazepines** – e.g. lorazepam, diazepam –
1. Both psychic and physical dependence occur.
2. **Clinical features of chronic benzodiazepine dependence** –
   a. Unsteadiness of gait.
   b. Dysarthria.
   c. Drowsiness.
   d. Nystagmus.
3. **Withdrawal effects from benzodiazepines** –
   a. Rebound insomnia; tremor.
   b. Anxiety; restlessness.
   c. Appetite disturbance; weight loss.
   d. Sweating; convulsions.
   e. Confusion; toxic psychosis.
   f. A condition resembling delirium tremens.

Aetiology

I. **Availability of drugs.**

II. **Vulnerable personality** –
1. People with personality disorder.
2. People from severely disorganized backgrounds, e.g. a history of childhood unhappiness.

III. **Social pressures** – for a young person to take drugs to achieve status, within the immediate peer group.

IV. **Pharmacological mechanisms** – suggestion that tolerance and physical withdrawal effects can be explained by –:
1. An increased neurotransmitter receptor supersensitivity.
2. Hypertrophy of alternative pathways.
3. Dysfunction of endorphin metabolism.

Management

I. **Physical** –
1. **Withdrawal effects from opiates** – two ways of treating –
   a. Methadone –
      i. Given as a linctus in a reducing dosage regime.
      ii. Undertaken as an out-patient or in-patient.
   b. Symptomatic relief – using chlorpromazine and analgesics.
2. **Withdrawal effects from barbiturates** –
   a. Dosage reduction of barbiturate.
   b. Cover withdrawal symptoms with a benzodiazepine.
   c. Use anticonvulsants if necessary.
   d. Nearly always undertaken as an inpatient.
3. **Withdrawal effects from benzodiazepines** –
   a. Switch from a short-acting benzodiazepine (e.g. lorazepam) to a long-acting (e.g. diazepam).
   b. Dosage reduction of benzodiazepine.
   c. Cover withdrawal symptoms with an antidepressant (e.g. dothiepin 150 mg nocte).
   d. Undertaken as an out-patient or in-patient.

II. **Social** –

Rehabilitation – the aim of this is to enable the addict to leave the drug subculture, and develop new social contacts, by way of:
1. The interest and support of a caring person.
2. Accommodation.
3. Work.

III. **Psychological** –

Group psychotherapy –
1. For patients with a vulnerable personality.
2. Used to help patients develop insight into their emotional and personality problems.
3. Group sessions involve intense confrontation with considerable emotional release.

CHAPTER 11

Psychiatric Emergencies

NON-FATAL DELIBERATE SELF-HARM (DSH)

I. **Definition** – a deliberate non-fatal act, whether physical, drug overdosage or poisoning, done in the knowledge that it was potentially harmful, and in the case of drug overdosage, that the amount taken was excessive.

II. **Motives** –

1. The wish to die.
2. 'A cry for help' – aimed at changing a seemingly intolerable situation.
3. An attempt to influence other(s) – e.g. seeking to make a relative feel guilty for failing the patient in some way.
4. Escape from emotional distress – the patient seeking immediate relief from his state of mind through temporary oblivion (i.e. unconsciousness).
5. Anger directed at a loved one – and sometimes redirected against the self.
6. Testing the benevolence of 'fate'.

III. **Significant predictors of serious suicidal risk in patients following DSH** –

1. **Circumstances suggesting high suicidal intent in the DSH act** –
    a. Planning in advance (i.e. premeditated).
    b. Precautions to avoid discovery.
    c. Carried out alone.
    d. No attempts to obtain help afterwards.
    e. Dangerous or violent method.
    f. 'Final acts' – e.g. suicide note or making a will.
2. **History of previous DSH.**
3. **Male sex.**
4. **Older age group (over 45 years old).**

5. **Psychiatric illness** –
   a. Depressive disorders.
   b. Alcohol or drug dependence.
   c. Antisocial personality disorder.
6. **Social isolation.**
7. **Unemployment.**

N.B. 10% of patients admitted to hospital following DSH commit suicide within ten years.

THE ACUTELY DISTURBED PATIENT

I. **Aetiology** –
   1. Alcohol or drug dependence.
   2. Prescribed drugs.
   3. Metabolic disturbance.
   4. Head injury.
   5. Schizophrenia.
   6. Mania.
   7. Personality disorders.

II. **Management** – acutely disturbed behaviour demands immediate action, often before the underlying cause has been determined.
   1. Much can be done by providing a calm, reassuring, and consistent environment in which provocation is avoided.
   2. A special ward area with an adequate number of experienced staff is much better than the use of heavy medication.
   3. However, physical restraint and medication is often needed to bring acutely disturbed behaviour under immediate control:
      a. Haloperidol is a better drug than chlorpromazine for this purpose, since haloperidol is less sedating, and causes less postural hypotension and fewer anticholinergic side-effects. However, it does have the disadvantage of causing more extrapyramidal side-effects.
      b. Up to 30 mg of haloperidol may be given intramuscularly in a single dose for emergency control.
      c. If haloperidol alone fails to bring the situation under control, the patient may be given in addition an intravenous injection of 4 mg of lorazepam.

THE MENTAL HEALTH ACT (MHA) 1983

I. **Use** –

1. With skill and patience, a sympathetic doctor can often persuade an initially uncooperative patient to accept hospital admission.
2. However, occasionally compulsory hospital admission and detention under the MHA 1983 will be required.

II. **Indications for compulsory admission and detention under the MHA 1983** –

1. The patient must suffer from a mental disorder of a nature and degree which warrants hospital detention for assessment or treatment –
   a. In the interests of his own health or safety.
   b. With a view to the protection of others.
2. There are four categories of mental disorder –
   a. Mental illness.
   b. Mental impairment.
   c. Severe mental impairment.
   d. Psychopathic disorder.
3. The following are not regarded as mental disorders and are therefore excluded from the MHA –
   a. Alcohol or drug dependence.
   b. Promiscuity or immoral conduct.
   c. Sexual deviancy.

II. **Admission for assessment** –

1. **Section 5(2)** –
   a. An order for the emergency detention of a patient who is already in hospital as a voluntary patient but wishes to leave.
   b. It requires a single medical recommendation by the doctor in charge of the case (i.e. the responsible medical officer) or his or her nominated deputee (i.e. the senior house officer or registrar in psychiatry).
   c. The duration of the section is 72 hours.
2. **Section 2** –
   a. An order for the compulsory admission of a patient when informal admission is not appropriate in the circumstances.
   b. Detention is for assessment, or for assessment followed by medical treatment.

c. It requires –
   i. Medical recommendation by two doctors, one of whom is a section 12 'approved doctor' (e.g. the senior registrar or consultant in psychiatry), the other who has preferably previous knowledge of the patient (e.g. the patient's general practitioner).
   ii. Application by the patient's nearest relative or an approved social worker.

d. The duration of the section is 28 days.

3. **Section 4** –
   a. An order for the compulsory detention of a patient in an emergency.
   b. It should be used only when there is insufficient time to obtain the opinion of a section 12 'approved doctor' who could complete section 2.
   c. It is usually completed in the patient's home by his or her general practitioner; it is occasionally used in the general hospital casualty department.
   d. It is expected that a section 4 order will be converted to a section 2 order as soon as possible after the patient has arrived in hospital.
   e. It requires –
      i. Medical recommendation by one doctor, who must have examined the patient within the previous 24 hours; he need not be a section 12 'approved doctor' (e.g. the patient's general practitioner, a senior house officer or registrar in psychiatry, a casualty officer).
      ii. Application by the patient's nearest relative or an approved social worker.
   f. The duration of the section is 72 hours.

IV. **Admission for treatment** –
Section 3 –
1. An order for the compulsory admission of a patient for treatment.
2. It requires –
   a. Medical recommendation as for section 2. It must specify –
      i. Which of the four categories of mental disorder the patient is suffering from.
      ii. Whether any other methods of dealing with the patient are available and, if so, why they are not appropriate.

   b. Application by the patient's nearest relative or an approved social worker.

3. The duration of the section is six months.